Bound by Numbers

Bound by Numbers

Abandoning the Control Weight has Over You

Angela Lutz

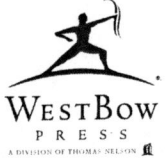

WestBow
PRESS
A DIVISION OF THOMAS NELSON

Copyright © 2012 Angela Lutz

All rights reserved. No part of this book may be used or reproduced by any means, graphic, electronic, or mechanical, including photocopying, recording, taping or by any information storage retrieval system without the written permission of the publisher except in the case of brief quotations embodied in critical articles and reviews.

Unless otherwise indicated, all scripture quotations are taken from the Message version of the bible. Copyright © 1954, 1958, 1962, 1964, 1965, 1987 by The Lockman Foundation. Used by permission. All rights reserved.

Scripture noted as NKJV taken from the New King James Version of the Bible. Copyright 1979, 1980, 1982 by Thomas Nelson, Inc. Used by permission. All rights reserved.

WestBow Press books may be ordered through booksellers or by contacting:

WestBow Press
A Division of Thomas Nelson
1663 Liberty Drive
Bloomington, IN 47403
www.westbowpress.com
1-(866) 928-1240

Because of the dynamic nature of the Internet, any web addresses or links contained in this book may have changed since publication and may no longer be valid. The views expressed in this work are solely those of the author and do not necessarily reflect the views of the publisher, and the publisher hereby disclaims any responsibility for them.

Any people depicted in stock imagery provided by Thinkstock are models, and such images are being used for illustrative purposes only.

Certain stock imagery © Thinkstock.

ISBN: 978-1-4497-4097-9 (sc)
ISBN: 978-1-4497-4098-6 (hc)
ISBN: 978-1-4497-4096-2 (e)

Library of Congress Control Number: 2012903192

Printed in the United States of America

WestBow Press rev. date: 3/4/2013

Contents

Acknowledgments ix
Introduction xi
Chapter 1. A Recounting of Devastation 1
Chapter 2. Going On 15
Chapter 3. Satan's Tool: Self-Sabotage 25
Chapter 4. What You Put in Your Mouth 31
Chapter 5. Reveal and Deal 39
Chapter 6. Self-Destructive Behavior: The Silent Sower ... 49
Chapter 7. Weeding Out Your Soul with Forgiveness 57
Chapter 8. Vital Vision 63
Chapter 9. Reevaluating Fixations 67
Chapter 10. Fueling the Vehicle of Your Soul 73
Chapter 11. Operation "Move It" 79
Chapter 12. Fruits of the Spirit 81
Chapter 13. Conclusion: Numbers Can Do a Number on Us ... 85
Notes 89

I dedicate this book to my mother, who was wise beyond her years. She celebrated life with a carefree spirit, transcending priceless lessons on life through her journey and departure. Her belief in me was unwavering as she showed me the importance of trusting myself.

I also dedicate this book to my daughter, who was a gift with perfect timing. Olivia's arrival flooded my world with hope and served as a reminder that every life (even my own) has a divine purpose. It is because of her that I have learned the importance of trusting others.

Acknowledgments

This project has not been a solitary effort. On the contrary, I have been blessed to have amazing people enter my life and support my vision. I gratefully acknowledge the contributions by those who have made the journey possible.

I have learned priceless lessons from so many of my clients as they walked out their own journey to freedom.

To those who have cheered me on in this endeavor—Tracy Cox, Tonda Moore, Ann Ritnour, and Jim and Beth Whittaker—I am honored to have you in my corner.

It takes a team to actually create a book, and I am thankful that my team included Jodi Hufschmitt's editing skills during the early stages of this manuscript; Deanna Stevens and her writing, coaching, editing, and creative vision in shaping this book for publication; and Brandon J. Schmidt, who designed the cover and poured countless hours into making this project a success.

A heartfelt thanks to Kevin Lafarriere for his inspiring instruction regarding all things pertaining to health, fitness, longevity, and relationship. His wisdom contributed to both my professional and personal success.

Of special note are my spiritual mentors: Pastors Gary and Drenda Keesee, Pastor Clyde and Scheherazade Daniels, Brother Chris D'Amico, and my Aunt Claire Gallagher, an amazing minister of God whose guidance, teachings, and impartations were critical in shaping me into the person I am today and inspiring me to do big things for my Lord and Savior, Jesus Christ.

I am deeply grateful to Kendra Flack—my forever friend and the boss of me. No matter the circumstance, she refused to allow my dream to become anything less than reality. Kendra, your loyal and steadfast friendship has been—and always will be—invaluable to me. Thank you for all your hard work and support.

Connie, God sure knew what He was doing when He placed you in my life when I was ten years old. You have been a constant source of encouragement and one of my biggest fans. Thank you.

To the little *great big loves* of my life—my daughter, Olivia, and my son, Angelo. Thanks for enduring countless Saturdays in your jammies so Mommy could write. You are an eternal source of inspiration. I am so honored to be your mom.

And finally to my soul mate, Esteban, for his love and undying commitment. Thank you for always believing in me and my dreams. I love you.

Introduction

The dreams, ideas, goals, and works God wants to create through us and in us are often so much more than we can comprehend in the natural world.

The very second this knowledge was revealed to me became a turning point. My life immediately underwent a drastic transformation as my outlook changed from hopelessness and fear into confidence and peace. I began to look at events differently; the future became something to joyfully anticipate. While I continue to grow, learn, and discover the vastness of God's love and mercy, each season supersedes the previous one, and I am beginning to understand the concept of going "from glory to glory" (2 Corinthians 3:18).

The Lord came to me in a prophetic dream in November 2005 and showed me a picture of a small group of women whom He was speaking to through me. In the dream, I was praying over these women using God's words, and the women were being healed of various afflictions. The dream was so real that I woke up feeling refreshed and on fire for what God had planned for me; at the same time, I was extremely confused. I knew that the dream was a representation of my future, but I had no idea what action I should take. I didn't know what to say or how to say it, nor could I fathom how any of it could possibly come to pass.

At the time I experienced the dream, the idea of praying over people and their being healed was not something I could even imagine. As a matter of fact, I was personally struggling through a series of difficult circumstances, and I needed all the prayers I could get. To put it bluntly, my life was a mess. I was addicted to Phentermine (a habit-forming prescription diet medication) which allowed this single mother to wake up at 4:00 each morning, not eat for the entire day, and still be filled with enough energy to work as a personal trainer and health and fitness educator late into the evening. Additionally, I carried weighty responsibilities as sole provider for my young daughter and, following a failed first marriage, I was struggling with trust issues. I was plowing through life with an "I'll take care of everything!" attitude, not allowing myself to slip into the vulnerable position of relying on anyone for anything.

As days passed, I continued to think about the dream and what it might mean, but after taking inventory of my life, it was painfully obvious that I needed to be standing in the prayer line instead of praying for others. My life was filled to capacity with many personal challenges. I was frank with God and let Him know that He had tapped the wrong individual for this mission. I began to list the many reasons I was definitely not the person for the job. Satisfied that I had successfully proven my case, I closed the door on the matter—or so I thought. Fortunately, God had other ideas for my future.

God simply wouldn't let me walk away from His mandate. During this time we engaged in several serious conversations, and He showed me how, because I was so wrapped up in my own kingdom, I couldn't even think about furthering His kingdom. Eventually, I came to realize the importance of thriving and living a healthy life in every area (physical, emotional, mental, and spiritual) so that I would be positioned to effectively demonstrate His works. Throughout our conversations, God began to impress upon me an urgency to take a thorough look at what was going on in my life. As I obediently followed His direction, the battle for freedom began.

I wrote *Bound by Numbers* as a spiritual approach to the individual battles our bodies and minds endure with image and weight. It was written specifically for *you*—because you are unique, and you were thoughtfully handcrafted by your Heavenly Father.

> *For You did form my inward parts; You did knit me together in my mother's womb. I will confess and praise You for You are fearful and*

wonderful and for the awful wonder of my birth! Wonderful are Your works, and that my inner self knows right well.

My frame was not hidden from You when I was being formed in secret [and] intricately and curiously wrought [as if embroidered with various colors] in the depths of the earth [a region of darkness and mystery]. Your eyes saw my unformed substance, and in Your book all the days [of my life] were written before ever they took shape, when as yet there was none of them.

Psalm 139:13–16

Take a minute to consider what this passage is telling you about your origins: knit in your mother's womb … the very hairs on your head were predetermined; you were intelligently designed and created purposely and purposefully—nothing was overlooked; every detail was designed down to the ridges on your fingertips and the freckles on your face. Before you were formed, God already had prepared a mission for you to accomplish. *You were thoughtfully planned by God for a definite purpose.*

God equipped you with physical characteristics that are uniquely yours. He thoughtfully created you with the intention to provide everything you would need to carry out your life's purpose. You have been ingrained with personal preferences to attract and be attracted by those God desires for you to intercept as you travel life's journey. There is a reason God created us as individuals—that no two people are identical. Your unique physical attributes were handcrafted by God to assist you in accomplishing His purpose. Your particular strengths, talents, and gifts were not bestowed for your own benefit. They were given so that you would be able to provide answers, assistance, and encouragement to others. You have been created in such a way as to appeal to those who require the inspiration you are able to provide.

God has crafted you specifically to distribute help and encouragement to others. Whether you are already aware of this truth or will come to realize it in the future makes no difference. God's divine destiny is to work through you for others. Only *you* can arrive at the precise time and place ordained for you to fulfill your responsibilities. There is no one else ordained to carry out your personal assignment. You—and you alone—have been created and prepared for this purpose.

> *Do you not know that your body is the temple [the very sanctuary] of the Holy Spirit who lives within you, whom you have received [as a gift] from God? You are not your own, you were bought with a price [purchased with a preciousness and paid for, made His own]. So then, honor God and bring glory to Him in your body.*
>
> 1 Corinthians 6:19–20

You are not your own. Your body is the armor that houses the most precious life force to ever exist on earth and in the heavens: your spirit, which is the very essence of your identity. You have been charged with a high calling and divine purpose; yours is not an errand to be taken lightly. Your purpose transcends far beyond the mere physicality of body image or a dissatisfying weight dilemma. The one true living God—the creator of the heavens and the earth—dwells in you. Every aspect of who you are is a representation of Him. Ultimately, you bear the responsibility for whether you allow others to witness His life moving through you or you obscure His image to others by promoting your own agenda and motives.

There is too much at stake, and you cannot afford to settle for anything less than God's very best. You must not allow overbooked calendars and out-of-control expectations to steal even one more precious second from your pursuit of God's plan for your life. Stop pushing aside your health in order to pursue your own visions and assignments. If you don't commit to maintaining good health, your vitality will drastically decrease, and you will fall far short of reaching your destiny. God created your body specifically for you and your ordained mission; your body is a temple, and keeping it in optimal condition must be a priority. What excuse could you possibly offer to God for failing to properly care for His creation, your body?

Unfortunately, when you arrived on earth, you were not handed an owner's manual with instructions on how to properly care for yourself.

Instead, facts, figures, studies, and reports have bombarded you from an assortment of sources with wildly varying ideas, viewpoints, and motives. So then, how can you possibly know the proper way to fulfill this great responsibility you have been given of caring for your body, the temple of the Holy Spirit?

I have written *Bound by Numbers* to present information that will challenge you to think consciously about the choices you make on a daily basis and how those choices ultimately affect your body, your family, and your future.

Remember, numbers are only a point of reference; their function is to indicate your position in place and time. You were never meant to build your life on a set of ever-changing numbers. Who you are cannot be interpreted through the sum of a few arbitrary digits. In grade school, the teachers called the process of manipulating numbers "problem solving." Perhaps that's where you obtained the inaccurate notion that you can look to numbers to solve your problems.

Authentic, permanent change cannot be charted on a graph; it originates from the inside and works toward the outside, and it takes time. First, seek healing for your heart. Then you will able to literally change your mind. Bear no unintended weight (guilt, shame, or contempt) emotionally, physically, or spiritually. Some days you're going to sleep in, skip the workout, and eat the pizza. That's okay! Realize that life is wonderfully imperfect. Embrace it! Enjoy it! Do not allow numbers to be a weapon. Put them in their proper place, and harness them as a tool for your benefit.

As you read through this book, my prayer is that you will be challenged to commit to a plan of action that will allow you to build a successful, positive, and abundant life. So, ready your armor for war and prepare to win a battle. Stand confident in the knowledge that no weapon used against you shall prosper, even if that weapon is *you*.

> *But no weapon that is formed against you shall prosper, and every tongue that shall rise against you in judgment you shall show to be in the wrong. This [peace, righteousness, security, triumph over opposition] is the heritage of the servants of the Lord [those in whom the ideal servant*

of the Lord is reproduced]; this is the righteousness or the vindication which they obtain from Me [this is that which I impart to them as their justification], says the Lord.

Isaiah 54:17

Your number is up. Let it go. Do not allow numbers to continue to dictate your outcome or maintain control over you. Numbers are wonderfully infinite, without end. Numbers are boundless in their infinite nature. They are limitless, endless, and inexhaustible. Indeed, you too are boundless in the very being of your own body. You have been unbounded by God's boundless love.

Chapter 1

A Recounting of Devastation

> *I do not consider, brethren, that I have captured and made it my own [yet]; but one thing I do [it is my one aspiration]: forgetting what lies behind and straining forward to what lies ahead, I press on toward the goal to win the [supreme and heavenly] prize to which God in Christ Jesus is calling us upward.*
>
> *So let those [of us] who are spiritually mature and full-grown have this mind and hold these convictions; and if in any respect you have a different attitude of mind, God will make that clear to you also.*
>
> Philippians 3:13–15

My breaking point occurred in 2003 during what should have been a wonderful season in my life: planning my wedding. After suffering through the devastation caused by my first husband's infidelity and the subsequent divorce, I had no intention of remarrying. However, I met Esteban at work, and he began to persistently and patiently pursue me. After several weeks of enduring my rebuffs, he finally convinced me to attend a Yankees game with him. He eventually won me over, and we dated for three years before deciding to wed.

Even with the arrival of such a kind and loving man in my life, I struggled with trust issues. I was working seven days a week, refusing to eat, exercising until I vomited, and continuing to take Phentermine, which I was addicted to. I was determined to do everything myself, including securing the finances for our wedding. I refused to allow Esteban to help in any way or pay for anything. To put it bluntly, I was suffering from fear of abandonment and didn't feel that I could risk depending on anyone for anything—not even my future husband. Unfortunately, this wasn't anything new for me. The theme of my life had been abandonment; it was woven throughout relationships: with my father, who left my mother on account of her infidelity before I turned three; with my mother, who died prematurely of cancer; with my brother, who took his own life; with my stepfather, who turned inward following my mother's death; and with my first husband, who engaged in an extramarital affair.

Driving my extreme behavior was an overwhelming desire for every detail of the wedding to be absolutely, unquestionably perfect. For me, this was more than a wedding; it was my chance for a new beginning. It was an opportunity for me to erase the failures and disappointments of my past. I desperately wanted to begin my life anew. I believed that, if I just worked hard enough and everything was perfect, I would be able to make amends for my past and walk down the aisle into a perfect future. Quite literally, however, I was working myself to death attempting to reach an impossible ideal.

Medication abuse, lack of eating, extreme exercising, and maintaining an impossible work schedule conspired to kill me, and I was rushed to the emergency room with severe chest pain. I weighed only eighty-nine pounds—far below a healthy weight for my five-foot, three-inch frame. The diagnosis included pericarditis (a viral infection of the heart), adrenal failure, and a potassium deficiency. During extensive testing at the hospital, a tumor was also discovered in my left breast.

Food had always been the one thing I could control in a world that was constantly out of control. My obsession with controlling food had evolved into the ultimate, extreme tactic of withholding food from myself altogether. Even though I couldn't see it at the time, I now realize that food had control of me, and my body was actually rotting from the inside out as I starved myself to death. This was not my first experience with anorexia nervosa—a disorder I began to battle following my mother's death in 1995—but it was the most severe. The trip to the hospital was a well-deserved slap in the face; a wake-up call if you will. My continuing battle with anorexia nervosa had resulted in a critical health crisis. I had been abusing my body by taking every diet pill ever created by man (both prescribed and over-the-counter), consuming no more than six hundred calories a day (which is equivalent to eating about three yogurts), and then exercising until I vomited.

I began working in the fitness industry in 1996, drawn to it because of its focus on health and wellness. I didn't realize it at the time, but I had chosen this path out of fear, a false sense of pride, and an attempt to assert self-control. It was a desperate attempt to prove to myself that I was "okay" and to validate my dreadful nutritional decisions. I became obsessed with learning all I could about the next "best" diet, and, in the process, I had accumulated an impressive collection of dieting books and resources. Unfortunately, amassing all the information in the world was ineffective at reversing the destruction caused by my harmful choices.

My hair was falling out of my scalp at an alarming rate. I developed unwanted facial hair, and my breath was rancid. I became dizzy every time I exercised or stood up too quickly. Nonetheless, I chose to ignore these and other signals that I was wasting away. Fueled by emotional stressors, I simply couldn't step off the destructive treadmill that held me captive. I was failing myself and my baby daughter, and I was a contradiction to everything I represented as a member of the health and fitness industry. I was broken, deceived, disillusioned, and living a life of denial and self-destruction.

It may sound strange, but when I looked in the mirror, it was actually easy to ignore all the frightening conditions reflected back at me. I could easily disregard reality and *see* what I wanted to see: a slim woman who was in control of her life. I wasn't able to see what was really going on inside of me or recognize how truly horrible I felt about myself and the inner struggles I battled every day. The mirror I looked into wasn't reflecting the truth; it was revealing a distorted image of the darkness that was trying to take control. My true reflection was revealed through my behavior and was completely unrelated to the image of the woman staring back at me from the mirror.

This duplicity is why we need to look to Christ as our standard; not to others, or even to ourselves. It wasn't until much later, when I made the decision to put Jesus "on" and began to wear the glory of God that I was able to see myself for who I truly was—an amazing creation thoughtfully designed by a loving Creator.

During this destructive period, I began to measure my self-worth by how little food I put into my body. And because I felt worthless, it felt good to withhold food and nutrients. Denying myself food validated my need to suffer for my unworthiness. I was convinced that my self-loathing was justified. I was a fake and a fraud, and my past was littered with selfish choices and more failures than I cared to remember.

I remember thinking that if I could just be disciplined and rigid enough, if I could just get it "right" and avoid making mistakes, I would eliminate the possibility of failure. I was willing, at any cost, to avoid the devastation that had destroyed my family and prevent it from pursuing me. I was confident that if I could just be perfect enough in every area of my life, I would be able to break free from the past that haunted me, free from the curse of being the cause and bearer of misfortune.

Satan knew that the joke was on me. The very thing I was running from was the very thing he was going to use to destroy me. I had watched my family suffer through fatal illness, debilitating health issues, divorce, abandonment, financial disasters, and suicide, and I thought I was being loyal by continuing to share in their misery. So began a warped and abusive relationship with food, as I accepted the spirit of drawn-out suffering, which is the belief that it was my responsibility to carry the weight of emotional pain and condemnation.

> *For we are not wrestling with flesh and blood [contending only with physical opponents], but against the despotisms, against the powers, against*

[the master spirits who are] the world rulers of this present darkness, against the spirit forces of wickedness in the heavenly [supernatural] sphere.

Ephesians 6:12

It is overwhelming to see how easily Satan, the father of lies, uses false realities to manipulate generations of families. If you believe you are destined to a life of interminable suffering, you are needlessly living in a false reality. You are trusting in the lies of one who wants to destroy you and your family instead of placing your confidence in Jesus: the One who willingly gave Himself for you. Jesus paid the ultimate price so you could enjoy a life of abundance, free from suffering, regardless of the circumstances you are facing.

But God—so rich is He in His Mercy! Because of and in order to satisfy the great and wonderful and intense love with which He loved us,

Even when we were dead [slain] by [our own] shortcomings and trespasses, He made us alive together in fellowship and in union with Christ; [He gave us the very life of Christ Himself, the same new life with which He quickened Him, for] it is by grace [His favor and Mercy which you did not deserve] that you are saved [delivered from judgment and made partakers of Christ's salvation].

Ephesians 2:4–5

Perhaps a little history is in order to explain how my hopelessness began and then how it spiraled out of control, creating a life-threatening health crisis and nearly resulting in my complete destruction.

I was raised in a Christian home, and from a young age, I had an awareness of God. Our family moved around from one church to another and, as a result, we attended Catholic, Baptist, Methodist, and nondenominational churches. By conventional standards, our spiritual education was unusual, as my siblings and I were encouraged to draw our own conclusions about religion.

While I experienced joy through the praise and worship songs my mom sang and played on her guitar, the idea of being in relationship with a God who is madly in love with me paled in comparison with the oppressive knowledge that, above all else, God's judgment was to be feared. I came to understand that Jesus had paid an enormous price and endured great suffering on my behalf through His crucifixion, and I should be willing to pay a great price to be considered His child. God's rules and punishments were clear, but little was spoken of the power of His love, grace, or healing.

Although my mother had made poor choices—which included two failed marriages—and endured a chaotic life as a result of her youthful decisions, she finally met her prince charming when I was in grade school. My stepfather was an amazing man who loved my mother and her children as his very own. He loved her free spirit and eccentric hippie worldview; they were a perfect match. But supporting our big blended family was a financial struggle and we often depended on welfare and food stamps.

No matter what our family was facing, I always knew that my mom loved her family more than anything, and I adored her! To me, she was perfection. My mom was my best friend and confidant. We had a very open relationship and I could (and did) discuss anything and everything with her. She patiently explained life choices and consequences, while trusting me to make the right decisions. I relied on her wisdom and followed her advice. I was a "good girl" who followed the rules—both God's and my mom's.

Despite her carefree attitude, my mom also held onto a lot of darkness and unforgiveness as a result of poor choices, broken relationships, and disappointments from her past. There were things she just couldn't forgive and forget. I now believe that the toxic emotions she couldn't escape festered in her spirit to the point of negatively impacting her physical health.

Shortly after I graduated from high school, my mother was diagnosed with stage-four lung cancer due, in no small part, to her smoking for years and aggravated, I believe, by the toxic emotional baggage she carried. By the time the doctors discovered the cancer, it had spread to her brain, and she was given six months to live. Not one to be swayed by bad news, my mother approached this situation like she did everything else—and carried on with a "whatever will be, will be" attitude. She accepted the illness simply for what she believed it was—the card she had been dealt in the game of her life. I thought God was using cancer to teach her a lesson or something—like, maybe, it was a message that she should quit smoking (which, by the way, she never did).

Mom didn't really discuss her illness with her family. True to form, she wanted to let reality be the teacher. She didn't call any family meetings. There weren't any big announcements. No plans were discussed for the future. "Que Sera Sera; Whatever Will Be Will Be" could have been her theme song.

I was aware my mom had cancer and that she had undergone surgery to remove the brain tumor, but I didn't have any idea that she might not survive, that this situation was something she might not be able to overcome. I was confident that she had everything under control and a plan to get healthy. Her plan was, "Let's see what happens."

One day, I recall entering her bedroom and asking, "Are you dying?"

She confirmed that she was, and when I pressed her to explain why she hadn't been more open with her diagnosis, her response was, "I wanted you to come to the conclusion yourself."

Chemotherapy left this once-vibrant woman sickly and without hair before the age of thirty-nine. I dropped out of college to help care for her, and I remember my routine consisting of waking each morning and checking to see if she had lived through the night. As I walked from my room to hers, I would make a declaration under my breath that I would never smoke and I would care for my body with the utmost of respect. *But isn't it just like Satan to use the very strength that drives you for his advantage and your destruction?*

Throughout my life, I had watched Mom struggle from one disappointment to another. From her finances to her relationships, and now, with her declining health, I had been a steadfast witness to her suffering. I watched as my best friend—my beloved mother—slowly deteriorated, struggled for her final breaths, and then slipped away as she lay in her bedroom. From the day cancer stole my mother from me, I vowed to be a crusader for life and vitality. Unfortunately, my plans veered wildly off track and gave way to years of self-destructive behavior.

My mom's cancer and subsequent death left me with more questions than answers. If her terminal illness was God's judgment on a loving mother and devoted wife—if her good works were ineffective against the curse of cancer—then what lesson was there for me to learn? I became convinced that following the rules and living a proper life didn't make any difference in the end. Why bother? I reasoned that, while I had been a "good girl" who followed the rules, my efforts had been in vain. I simply couldn't live a life good enough to avoid the tragedy of losing my mother at such a young age.

The very core of my belief system had been shaken, and Satan took advantage of my confusion. During this time, fear became the driving force that motivated my decisions and manipulated the choices I made about food. I may have been unable to control the results of my good works, but I could definitely control what I put into my body. Looking back, I can see that I was desperate for any answer that would help me avoid the catastrophic life my mother had endured. *Save yourself at any cost!* became my battle cry.

Satan's manipulation of my thoughts, ideas, and actions was insidious. As I immersed myself in class after class on holistic health and nutrition, I began obsessing over every chemical component in food. I studied the manner in which ingredients become altered during absorption and delivery as they enter the body's digestive system. The Bible says that God's people perish for lack of knowledge (Hosea 4:6), but there is a very fine line between knowledge and bondage, especially when you have allowed an idea to take over your life. I was obsessive, taking this newfound knowledge to the extreme, as I allowed food to dictate my behavior. I permitted food (or the lack thereof) to become the complete and final authority over my body image. This thinking eventually led to an unhealthy fear of food and an overwhelming anxiety every time I sat down to eat.

Fanatically, I endorsed our panic-stricken society's ideals regarding health and weight management. At the time, I didn't understand the dangers of using these ideals as a standard, and, as I looked to the world for answers, I walked away with a warped perspective of truth. I became consumed with the fear of retaining or gaining a calorie, an inch, a pound, or a size; the mere whisper of an increase sent me over the edge.

The type of fear I experienced is quite dangerous, as it generates an unhealthy attitude toward food and often results in binging, purging, overeating, or the withdrawal of food altogether. Do not be deceived; when an action is motivated by fear, the result is dysfunction.

Over time, I arrived at the realization that the issue wasn't the food at all; it was my faith.

When we are operating in the realm of human physicality, we might encounter an opposition to our faith that is not initiated by God. We are born into a physical world, one filled with sin and weakness and corruption. The earth is Satan's territory, and he persistently attempts to lead us down a path where we begin to see the body as our enemy, instead of as a chosen vessel crafted by a loving Creator for a divine purpose.

Whether a person is over-consuming or under-consuming food, Satan's emotionally-induced deception requires the abandonment of our rightful authority; the surrender of jurisdiction over our minds. He slowly destroys, insinuating the belief that the body is disgusting; as a person accepts this lie, he or she might begin to eat in secret to fill up the dark spaces in the heart. This creates a devoid—an emptiness—because something (the authority God gave all of us) has been relinquished. Satan then has freedom to move in and establish his own agenda. He does his damndest to take away the abundant life God has provided by turning us against ourselves.

You must take a stand against Satan's destructive plans and reclaim the God-given authority over your body and your mind.

You must also repent for allowing food to have the final authority and then restore Jesus as the Lord of your life so He has the sovereign access He needs to work on your behalf. Just as you don't heal apart from Jesus, you should not eat apart from Him either. If you don't stand against these controlling spirits from the moment they begin whispering their deceitful ideas, you will eventually arrive at the end of your will power and, often without even realizing it, submissively enter into an abusive relationship with food. In the process, you will have promoted food from nutrients created to serve you to an authority wielding power over you.

When you consistently eat too much or too little, you have given complete control to the food itself, allowing it to dictate how you feel. The food alone—whether a carbohydrate, protein, or fat—is not a magic ingredient that will repair the issues you have with your weight.

It's time to ask yourself some difficult questions:
- What drives your food choices right now?
- Do you eat with reckless abandon?
- Are you driven by fear? Or is your eating motivated by God?
- Do you realize that what you put into your body—or what you avoid—affects your ability to hear the voice of the Holy Spirit?

Before you try another fad diet and do something unhealthy (like deprive your body of carbohydrates), have you asked the One who created you whether or not your plan is His desire? Before you commit to doing whatever is necessary to fit into a size two, have you even stopped to ask your Creator if He created you to be a size two? Have you ever had a discussion with your Heavenly Father about your weight, your size, or your dietary needs? Do you know what He designed for you? Are you willing to commit to His course of action?

Are you overwhelmed when choosing foods? Are your self-imposed limitations and restrictions choking your ability to enjoy food? Are your choices influenced by fear of the consequences your psyche will suffer?

Do you have the food or does the food have you?

When dread drives your choices, you reap decay. When you exclude God and attempt to tackle food issues without Him, you have invited bondage—enslavement, if you will—into your life. God cannot identify with your choice of imprisonment, as these choices are not of Him. Are you comfortable participating in activities that exclude God?

You cannot afford to continue allowing food to dictate whether you reach your ideal physical potential. The time has come for you to take authority over the abusive relationship you have with food and return the control to your Lord and Savior, as Jesus directed:

> *I will give you the keys of the kingdom of heaven; and whatever you bind [declare to be improper and unlawful] on earth must be what is already bound in heaven; and whatever you loose [declare lawful] on earth must be what is already loosed in heaven.*
>
> Matthew 16:19

I invite you to pray this prayer with me:

> *Lord Jesus, I bind the controlling spirit of food from my presence. I pray that fear no longer has the power to paralyze or dictate my choices. By the authority given to me through Christ Jesus, I declare this spirit of control to be banished from my life.*

Jesus assures us in John 14:13 that He will grant whatever we ask of our Heavenly Father in His name. He also promises us in Luke 10:19 that "nothing by any means shall harm us." It is your God-given birthright to safely trample on serpents and scorpions whether they threaten you physically or torment you mentally. You possess the keys to God's kingdom and have been given divine authority over the works of the enemy. This includes taking authority over the food issues Satan has been using to torture you.

This is where the true freedom resides, my friends. Freedom is when you can walk in victory so that the choices you make about food do not originate from the food itself, nor do they come from the deeply rooted, multilayered beliefs you have accumulated about food; they are not created as a result of what others may have negatively sown into your subconscious. When you begin operating in your God-given authority, you are able to make proper choices about food by utilizing the knowledge He provides. At the same time, you can rest securely in the fact that God wants you to achieve your very best physical self and grow into your spiritual potential.

Soul Inceptions

When my motive is fear, the result is dysfunction.

Is fear the driving force that manipulates the choices I make about food?

Am I afraid of falling short and failing?

Have I allowed food to be the final authority in determining my body image issues?

Have I abandoned mental jurisdiction over my own emotions?

Chapter 2

Going On

After my mom passed away, darkness began to encompass me and, at nineteen years old, I felt my life started spinning out of control. Although I had been a "good girl"—I had followed the rules and lived a chaste life up to the point of my mother's death—I no longer saw the benefit of these choices. I sought men's attention to fill the dark void that had developed deep in the pit of my soul. I became involved in promiscuous relationships and began regularly smoking pot and drinking. My stepfather, struggling with his own grief, couldn't deal with my emotional breakdown, and we agreed that I needed to find a new place to live.

I became an exotic dancer at a local strip club. I was living on my own for the first time and had become responsible for paying my own way, and I rationalized my decision for the quick money it offered. Nevertheless, feelings of worthlessness consumed me.

My poor decisions had created distance between my stepfather, my siblings, and myself—my once-supportive family was a distant memory. I was disappointed in the person I was becoming. My actions weren't reflective of how I was raised. Exotic dancing, drinking, taking drugs—this wasn't the real me. Overwhelmed with regret and shame, I decided to take my own life. I consumed an entire bottle of prescription antidepressants, only to end up in the hospital getting my stomach pumped. One bad decision after another led me down the path toward destruction and heartbreak.

One evening, while I was getting high at my boyfriend's house, I had a vision of my mother. I clearly heard her speak in a firm voice of correction. *What are you doing to yourself? This is not who I raised you to be!*

Although I didn't realize it at the time, I now believe that this was the Holy Spirit attempting to get my attention. My drug-induced high came to an abrupt end, as did my craving for marijuana. With a newly clear mind, I looked around at my life, but all I could see was the mess I had created.

I was at the end of my rope when I called my stepmother for help. Connie had always been a supportive and positive influence, and during this time, she was living in New York with my biological father. (My father had walked away, very hurt from his marriage to my mom, when I was quite young. At the time, I had not yet developed the healthy relationship my dad and I now share.) After I shared with her everything that was going on in my life, Connie encouraged me to move in with her and my dad. I collected myself and relocated to New York where, after encouragement from a professor, I applied for and was awarded a scholarship to attend New York University's drama program.

Living in New York was a positive experience for me. I was able to put previous mistakes and disappointments firmly in the past as I moved forward with my life. I was attending college, having fun, and enjoying the love and support of family and friends. To my delight, I was also awarded several acting jobs. During my pursuit of work on Broadway, I was introduced to a family friend, and we began dating. During our courtship, he was very good to me, often bringing me flowers and taking me to the theater. Our relationship continued to grow and we eventually became engaged. Life was good ... for a season.

Six months before my wedding, my fourteen-year-old brother ended his life by putting a gun to his head in the bathroom of our family home. It had been four years since my mother had died, and the past came flooding back in a torrent. I felt that I had failed my brother. Following my mother's death, I should have acted as her surrogate and cared for my brother—instead of looking out for myself. Furthermore, I felt guilty, as I believed that my decisions, including "abandoning" my loved ones to move to New York and pursue my own life, had contributed to his death. Robert's suicide devastated my family—each one of us siblings carried a unique portion of the weight, blame, and responsibility for our youngest brother's death. I suffered constant torment as I watched the lives of my siblings slowly deteriorate after Robert's suicide. My stepfather became consumed with overwhelming grief that resulted in his suffering a series of strokes, leaving him unable to read, write, or speak.

Six months after my brother's death, I married; six months later, we conceived our daughter. I was just entering the third trimester of my pregnancy when things became uneasy in our marriage. I began to find tubes of lipstick and other feminine articles strategically hidden beneath the seats of our car. My husband's late-night phone calls, as well as the unusual breakfast and dinner charges that had begun appearing on credit card statements, forced my mind to accept what my heart wanted to ignore: there was someone else. When I questioned my husband, he denied the accusations and made me out to be a crazy pregnant woman. He vainly attempted to convince me that the lipstick I found was my own. But *Passion Pink* was never a part of my vocabulary, let alone my makeup case. The ugly truth was that my husband had become involved with another woman during the final months of my pregnancy.

I was suddenly facing divorce and the anguish of exchanging the joy of motherhood for the money a career could provide. I haphazardly began balancing competing priorities as I once again found myself on my own, but this time with the added responsibility of a new baby. I called Connie, who by this time had retired and relocated to Florida with my dad, and explained my situation. Again, she extended her offer of a home and encouraged me to bring my daughter and move in with them. I relocated to Florida and threw myself into a career within the health and fitness industry with the dream of creating a life for the new love of my life—my baby girl, Olivia.

Shortly after I arrived in Florida, I began attending Victorious Life Church, and I experienced God in a way that profoundly changed everything. VLC was my first introduction to a spirit-filled congregation, and I immediately connected with the enthusiasm, joy, and freedom of worship. I could tell the people were completely in love with God, and He loved them right back. I was so excited by what I was experiencing that I could barely sit still in that first service as I encountered God on an entirely new level. I came to the realization that I could trust God, and I made a vow that as long as I had God and the Holy Spirit in my life, Olivia and I certainly didn't need to depend on any man.

At work, my days were filled with managing the personal training team at Lifestyle Family Fitness, coaching on nutrition, educating personal trainers, teaching fitness classes, and serving my own personal training clientele. I conditioned myself to measure my worth by my performance, and seventy-hour work weeks became the norm. My hard work paid off as my club was often recognized as number one, and I enjoyed professional success while regularly meeting and exceeding my goals. As I worked my way up the corporate ladder, I was offered a management position, and I felt good about myself and my accomplishments for a change.

During this time, I was regularly attending church at VLC and continued to grow in grace and abound in the knowledge of God; He was transforming me into a healthy person. But the healing process took time, and it didn't come about quickly or without a fight. Keeping extremely busy allowed me to brush aside the huge, hurting void in my heart and played a large part in helping me ignore my disappointing past, my unhappy present, and how unworthy, undeserving, and ripped up I felt inside.

It is easy to become lost in your daily agendas. It is even easier to become consumed with your "To Do" list to the point where you begin to rationalize that, in the name of servitude, everything else should take priority over your well-being. You begin to feel justified putting your name last on the list and, before you know it, "I just don't have the time" is the excuse you employ for neglecting to take proper care of your physical, mental, and spiritual health.

Benjamin Franklin said, "He that is good for making excuses is seldom good for anything else."[1] What we often neglect to realize is that this principle has ramifications far beyond offering simple excuses. The danger is hidden in the fact that sometimes what we call an excuse is really an outright deception.

If you have ever said that you do not have the time to obtain a healthy body (which could mean freeing yourself from excess weight, gaining weight, or obtaining healing in your body), you have balance and priority issues and you are dealing with a spirit of distraction. If Satan can convince you that you do not have the time for yourself—to do what it takes to achieve a body of excellence—he is truly convincing you that you are unworthy of the time it will take to accomplish it. He'll make sure everything else takes priority, and you will follow his lead because, subconsciously, you will find it easier to cover up feelings of hurt and worthlessness with works and acts of service than to deal with the real issue. I am a living testimony to the fact that what you do not deal with on the inside will eventually reveal itself on the outside. The hope in this statement is that it works both ways: when you do deal with the inside, it's visible on the outside.

As 1 John 3:1 says, "Behold what manner of love the Father has bestowed on us, that we should be called children of God."

Know this: you are *not* what you do, your identity is secured through your relationship with God. However, in the name of ignoring and covering up what is really going on inside, you may have mistakenly allowed yourself to become identified with your packed schedule, important responsibilities, and acts of service.

You have been charged with a great responsibility. You have been blessed with certain talents, skills, and strengths that enable you to reach out to other people, gain access, be a support, answer a question, or unlock a revelation. Your skills were established by God so that, when opportunities arise to provide assistance at home or in the classroom or on the job, you show up wearing the characteristics of Christ. (In Ephesians 2:10, we learn that we are God's workmanship, created in Christ Jesus for good works.)

I wonder how Jesus must feel when He hears you say you're too busy and just don't have the time to put Him first. Why do you selfishly insist on doing things your own way? How can you blatantly reject His plan for your body—the very body He created for you? You are a masterpiece and His greatest work!

You must be available in your mind, your body, and your spirit to allow God to work and move through you. What good are you to Christ, your family, your friends, or the world if you can't think or act beyond your own self? What difference can you possibly hope to make if you are constantly consumed with your weight or you are wasting enormous amounts of time attempting to manage the destructive behaviors that torment you as a result of neglecting to take proper care of yourself?

Lying in that hospital bed, suffering from pericarditis, adrenal failure, and a potassium deficiency, I realized Satan had seized an opportunity to take advantage of my weaknesses when I was most vulnerable. Simply put, his desire was to destroy me. My insane work schedule, combined with an inability to trust, a desperate need for control and perfection, and feelings of not measuring up, had caused me to spiral downward into my worst and final episode of anorexia nervosa.

I began to desperately pray for my life: "Jesus, please save me from myself." For the very first time, I could see the truth of what was really happening to me and how my actions were affecting those I loved. It was a wake-up call with serious implications. If I didn't change my behavior, I would subject my young daughter to watching me slowly die, in the same way I had watched my own mother die.

I knew that I needed answers, and I was desperate to find them. A few weeks after my hospitalization, the Lord led me to attend a women's conference taking place in my home church. That night, Jesus revealed Himself to me in a powerful way. I received the Holy Spirit, and my life has never been the same. I was set free from the captivity of my physical body and from the generational curse of self-destructive behavior. I was also set free from the fear of death.

Jesus made a promise to me that night. As I lay in the awesome power of His presence at the altar, He vowed to engulf every inch of me with His love and give me the tools I needed to turn my life around. When I could finally stand, the ushers had to escort me back to my seat. My legs wobbled like those of a newborn fawn, but I was filled with confidence at the birth of my new life.

Once I was able to totally submit to Jesus and trust His plan for my life, I began a journey of divine healing. Along the way, there were times I received direct instruction from God. During other periods, I gained revelation and wisdom as a result of devotedly walking in obedience and faith. God is no respecter of persons; what He did for me He will do for you.

For God shows no partiality [undue favor or unfairness; with Him one man is not different from another].

Romans 2:11

It was like an avalanche of knowledge; large quantities of revelation were imparted to me, and I began to clearly see through the eyes of my Savior instead of peering through the cloudy glasses of my own humanity. I identified the spirit of drawn-out suffering that had held me captive, and I was able to grasp hold of freedom as the wisdom of God came flooding into my life. During this time, the Holy Spirit spoke into my heart:

From the time you were a very little girl, you watched your mom sacrifice and lay down her life for her children. You saw as her relationships mistreated her, and you watched how she sought to shelter you from pain. She gave you the very best she could. You watched her endure pain and hardships. She was so precious and beautiful to you as you saw the sacrifices she made on your behalf—a mother's love for her daughter. She lived a difficult life; nonetheless, she did her best to make it beautiful for her family.

After seeing her struggle through two failed marriages, you watched her fall in love and marry the man of her dreams—finally reaching a place of rest and happiness, only to discover that the suffering she endured had taken root, developing into tumors on her brain and a death sentence.

The spirit of drawn-out suffering started to speak to you and it questioned, "Why should your life be any different than her life? After all, you witnessed her sacrifice and suffering. Why should you be given the opportunity to live and thrive when you watched the very woman who had given birth to you slip away so unfairly?" The spirit of drawn-out suffering began to tell you that you did not deserve more out of life than your own mother had received.

On a subconscious level, you began to believe it would be unfair if you didn't endure suffering. By avoiding disaster, you believed you would lose any connection or identification that remained with her. Moreover, you became convinced that your happiness would be an act of utter betrayal toward those in your family who were barely sustaining their own lives. Doubt gave birth, and you questioned your right to succeed in life while the lives of your stepfather and siblings continued to deteriorate. Satan went to work on your vulnerabilities. He targeted your body and convinced you to carry out the destructive work for him. He continued to bombard your mind: "Why do you deserve to prosper in all areas of your life, when your mother did not? What gives you the authority to breathe if your brother is dead?

Like I had, many of you have simply stopped living. You continue to bear the dead weight of a precious life, someone who has gone from you before his or her time. You literally carry the weight upon your back and refuse relief from stress. This heavy burden manifests physically and reveals itself in your body as you remain loyal to suffering. You are desperate for a connection. In fact, you are so loyal that you verbally confess that the days of your life will not exceed the number of days your loved one lived.

You might even go as far as to plan your life around this loyalty and prepare your spouse for its eventuality. You jokingly caution that you will be looking down on him from heaven if he remarries too quickly. Be mindful of your conversation! Life and death, my friend, can be found in your tongue. You wonder why you struggle with your health and why your battle with weight feels like an endless roller-coaster ride, all the while speaking negatively of yourself and giving death a formal invitation to dinner.

You have the right to stop the influence of the spirit of drawn-out suffering in your life. It is my assignment to tell you that Satan has no choice but to bow to your authority when you exercise your rights. If you are battling the spirit of drawn-out suffering, I encourage you to declare the following over your life:

By the authority given to me in Christ Jesus—who endured the greatest of sufferings so I could live without them—I bind the spirit of drawn-out suffering and render it powerless in my life. I release healing so it may come into my heart and heal this area of my life.

Don't think that you have to address this issue on your own. I want to share a message Jesus has for you.

You are so beautiful to me. I have died to give you freedom, and it is time to receive it. The spirit of drawn-out suffering has been called out and identified. Devouring and sabotage stops here; I will allow no more!

That night at the women's conference, Jesus made it clear that I had responsibilities to meet if I desired to see the fulfillment of His promises in my life. I wrote *Bound by Numbers* to examine the steps I traveled on my road to recovery, as well as to arm you with the knowledge I have gained over the past eleven years regarding health and nutrition. I share this information with you in the hope that you may be set free from the battle with your body image and weight. I also want to make it clear that it is one thing to feel the hand of the Holy Spirit free you from captivity and quite another to embody that anointing in this natural world. To hear God's word and receive it is to be blessed. To act on His word is to watch miracles unfold before you.

But He said to me, "My grace [My favor and loving-kindness and mercy] is enough for you [sufficient against any danger and enables you to bear the trouble manfully]; for my strength and power are made perfect [is fulfilled and completed] and show themselves most effective in [your] weakness. Therefore, I will all the more gladly glory in my weaknesses and infirmities, that the strength and power of Christ [the Messiah] may rest [yes, may pitch a tent over and dwell] upon me.

2 Corinthians 12:9

Soul Inceptions

If Satan can convince you that you do not have the time to achieve a body of excellence, you are allowing him to convince you that you are unworthy.

You are not what you do. Your identity is rooted in Christ, not determined by your actions. Do not grant works and busyness the permission to steal your identity or distract you from the issues you need to address.

What good are you to others if you remain consumed with your weight and the destructive symptoms that occur when you neglect to take proper care of yourself?

Identify and stand against the devouring tactics the spirit of drawn-out suffering has over your body.

Chapter 3

Satan's Tool: Self-Sabotage

Satan is very strategic in creating destruction and diversions to sabotage you. Yo-yo dieting, overeating, compulsive eating, emotionally-induced eating, bulimia, anorexia nervosa, obesity, disorderly eating, diet pills, diuretics, quick-fix weight loss, and diet fads are all tools that he uses to paralyze you and keep you from walking out God's glory and purpose for your life.

More than 64 percent of people living in the United States are overweight, and approximately 33 percent of those overweight adults are estimated to be obese.[1] Even more alarming is the fact that twelve- to nineteen-year-olds are the fastest growing segment of the population of obese people in the United States.[2]

According to the National Association of Anorexia Nervosa and Associated Disorders, eating disorders have reached an all-time high in America, affecting seven million women and one million men. One out of three dieters develops compulsive dieting behaviors and unhealthy attitudes towards body image and food.[3]

Advertising and media industries vomit out garbage nonstop, giving us visual cues regarding what "good" looks like. Billboards, television programs, movies, and magazines promote images of women and supermodels with young, boyish, airbrushed figures sporting plastic body parts. Women are constantly instructed on how to look—force-fed an ideal that is neither easily obtainable nor healthy. Our society has become obsessed with meeting the expectations and standards of unspoken subliminal messaging, striving for approval from the land of make-believe—not to achieve personal happiness, but to appease "them." Collectively, we have bought into the belief that satisfying *their* requirements will cause us to feel better about ourselves. We adopt the form of an externalized object trying to please a counterfeit god. We are being used.

The economy generates millions of dollars from consumers while distorting the concept of how a healthy person should appear. Industry leaders do not think about the consequences of their actions (other than the resulting profit) or how their decisions affect people on an individual level, nor do they care. In response, Americans spend an estimated average of $46 billion per year on dieting and diet-related products, keeping the industry going strong.[4]

We have an entire segment of society chasing after an unobtainable, unhealthy image and throwing money away on the next quick fix with an "all or nothing" attitude. And, when the unrealistic diet or exercise program fails, the vicious cycle begins anew. Self-condemnation, as well as blaming others, becomes common behavior in a "justifiable search" of the ultimate prize: society's artificially designed woman.

Satan's goal is to cause you to personally struggle to attain this counterfeit female standard, creating conflict between individual women in the process. Let's discuss one very familiar strategy: The Look. It's that head-to-toe thing you do to other women with your eyes when you compare and condemn. The enemy knows that if he can keep you from blessing that to which you aspire, he can sabotage your efforts and keep you confined within the captivity of your body. Statistics prove that it only takes about eleven seconds to make a first impression.[5] This means it only takes eleven seconds to make a significant number of judgments about a woman whom you have just met.

You can never really be who God created you to be—nor can you celebrate the way He formed and designed your body—if you are relying on the false beliefs and perceptions you have developed as a result of comparing yourself to others. Furthermore, you cannot succeed in obtaining a body of excellence when you are constantly comparing and condemning. The Bible says that when you condemn, you can expect to receive condemnation in return.

> *Judge not [neither pronouncing judgment nor subjecting to censure], and you will not be judged; do not condemn and pronounce guilty, and you will not be condemned and pronounced guilty; acquit and forgive and release [give up resentment, let it drop], and you will be acquitted and forgiven and released.*
>
> Luke 6:37

When you constantly compare yourself to others (and pick yourself apart in the process), you choke out the ability for anything other than condemnation to grow. Who you really are is who you are in Christ. Your beliefs and perceptions should only come from what His word says about you, and His word, in Genesis 1:27, says that we are made in His image.

When you look in the mirror, who is looking back at you? The reflection you should see is your own. All too often, however, you see a mosaic of various sources inspecting you with unspoken—yet very loud—expectations. Remember this: You are *you*; you are not *them*. This journey is between you and God—not between you and them.

When you give love, you receive love in return; when you give compliments, you receive compliments in return. It's not a secret that you receive what you give. Don't overlook the mechanics of this principle: In order to receive, you must give. Action is required on your part. If you put good stuff in your life, good stuff will come out, and it will be evident to others. What you focus on and what you give awareness to is what you become.

I would like to share an example about the dangers of listening to *them* and comparing yourself to others. In January 2006, I met with a client who was determined to make a life change once and for all. During our consultation, she slid an old photo of herself—a picture of her in her twenties—across the desk, pointed to the image, and stated that this was her ultimate goal.

God began to speak to me, and He brought to mind every client who had ever handed me an old photo of herself, aspiring to look just as she had "back then." He reminded me that, once you are made new in Christ, there is no going back to your former self. In other words, you cannot compare yourself with anyone, not even with a younger version of yourself.

Let's suppose the "thin" dream girl featured in the old photo was an unhappy newlywed suffering with low self-esteem because her husband was addicted to pornography. She attempted to console herself through shopping and, in the process, accumulated a massive amount of credit card debt. Let's also assume that, during the first three years of marriage, this woman fought hard to save the relationship. As a result, she had collected an impressive number of emotional scars. In desperation, the couple turned to God. He faithfully began to restore and heal their marriage, and soon they were thrilled with the news of her pregnancy. Nine months and ninety-two pounds later, the wife delivered a beautiful baby boy. Their new son completed the family's union in ecstatic wholeness.

My client's attempt to return to that image of the girl in her past meant recalling all the former hurts she had endured. Subconsciously, she feared a repeat of past events. Furthermore, and even deeper-rooted still, was the belief that shedding the pregnancy weight might mean destroying the newly restored relationship with her husband. Even though she didn't realize it, the weight gain corresponded to a very happy time in her life. Inherently, the struggle she would face with her weight would always be present—as long as she desired to return to the woman of her past. The "thin" image of herself represented a certain place in her history and everything associated with it, not just the shape of her body at that time.

Many of you are also desperately attempting to hold on to the girl of yesteryear, not realizing that you are allowing her to keep you from attaining what you desire. It is time to release your former self and embrace the you who has been made a new creature in Christ.

Once you enter into a relationship with Jesus, you begin to mature in Him, and, during the process, you become an amazingly better version of who you once were. You can no longer return to your former self—spiritually or physically—because it is against God's nature. And, because you are becoming more and more like Him, it is against your new nature as well. The future God has for you is far better than anything you can dig up from the past. Begin to accept God's plan, and visualize a detailed version of yourself in the body of excellence He designed with beauty and splendor just for you.

Soul Inceptions

You cannot succeed in obtaining a body of excellence when you are constantly comparing yourself to others.

You cannot compare yourself even to your past self.

Chapter 4

What You Put in Your Mouth

Think back to the last time you visited the local shopping mall. Imagine sitting in the shoe department and trying on a pair of shoes that catches your attention. Next to you, an attractive stranger takes a seat, and, as you discreetly look her over, an internal dialogue begins. You notice that her hips are much narrower, her legs longer, and her tummy flatter than your own. However, the judgment doesn't stop with her physical appearance; you also begin to judge her inner being. In the process, you develop beliefs about what type of person "a woman who looks like that," really is.

Be careful. This is an intricate trap set for you by the enemy, and it works something like this: The next time you embark on the a new diet program, your subconscious will begin feeding you ideas in an attempt to sabotage your efforts to reclaim the "good-looking" body you desire. The very words and thoughts you have projected toward those attractive strangers become manifested in what you now think about the body you are trying to attain. And because you would never want to become a self-centered, egotistical, self-righteous—*feel free to fill in the blank*—"attractive stranger," your subconscious undermines your progress, until one day, you realize that the thirty pounds you had worked so hard to lose have returned.

This same scenario plays out again and again in many different circumstances. You may have a slim frame and project judgmental thoughts and attitudes toward overweight strangers. During your efforts to eat properly and maintain a healthy weight, the words and thoughts you have projected on those "unattractive strangers" become manifested in what you now think about the body you are trying to attain. And because you would never want to become a lazy, out-of-shape, offensive—*again, feel free to fill in the blank*—"unattractive stranger," your subconscious undermines your progress, until one day you realize that you are suffering with anorexia nervosa because food has lost its appeal.

These are just two examples of ways that Satan can establish a stronghold in your life. Thoughts are powerful, and your own words can be the very weapon the enemy uses against you. Working together, your mind and mouth have the ability to advance, hinder, or halt your progress altogether.

Fashion and glamour magazines can also trip you up. As you flip from page to page and see one beautiful model after another, the process begins again. You murmur and think to yourself, *They may be attractive, but they probably look that way because they are conceited and don't eat. They take drugs, spend all their money on personal trainers, and, most likely, employ full-time chefs.* You call them ugly names and—even worse—confess with your mouth that you could never look *that* beautiful. After all, your mind tells you, the woman in the photo must have been manufactured by a team of professionals because she has money, staff, opportunities, and a supply of never-ending resources that aren't available to you.

Here you go again, traveling down a road with a predictable destination. As you work to lose five, ten, or fifteen pounds and you get closer to that "ideal image," POW! Your subconscious suddenly remembers what you said about those fashion models: *To achieve success, you need a full-time chef and a personal trainer, and you have to starve yourself. Those models are self-indulged, pampered, nasty people.* And since *you* are not a nasty person, nor do you employ a full-time chef and a personal trainer, you unknowingly sabotage your progress. You begin to think, *What's the use? This never works for me! I might as well just give up!* You find yourself right back where you started.

Recently, I observed this play out in an airport. I was returning to Columbus after teaching an assessment seminar in Florida, and I had forty-five minutes to grab a bite to eat before my plane was scheduled to begin boarding.

As I sat down at the table in a restaurant, I noticed an older woman seated several tables away who was exhibiting signs of food stress. (The signs can be obvious or barely noticeable; sometimes they are recognizable by how much fussing a person makes over the menu or how many special requests are made for *this item* on the side or to substitute *that item* or make sure *none of that* is on the plate.) From her actions and conversation, it became clear to me that this woman had been battling with her weight. I also could see that the target of her immediate attention was a young, attractively slender woman who was sitting near me.

The younger woman was, in fact, beautiful. She was tall, slender, and very well dressed. She had taken care to match her handbag to her shoes; her jewelry tastefully suited her designer apparel. Throughout her meal, the older woman intermittently turned to her traveling companions to make disparaging comments about the young woman and snide remarks about her order.

I sat back and watched as the older woman lost forty-five minutes of her life, as well as the battle for her own self-image, while she verbally attacked the younger woman. I could visualize the trash floating around her mind. Instead of enjoying a pleasant dinner with loved ones, the older woman had foolishly squandered her time and sabotaged her future.

Strangely enough, I observed the younger, well-dressed woman round her shoulders into her chest and lower her head as she hovered over her plate of food. She clearly also felt uncomfortable throughout the meal. It appeared to me that there may have been some food stress going on at her table, too.

As a woman, you have a responsibility to think and speak blessings over the lives of your sisters. Recognize that while Satan does his best to stop you from imparting your love, wisdom, and support to one another, God's will is for you to love—and love, and love. You are to love profoundly in order to stamp out all insecurity. Love is the only way to break through the gates of self-sabotage and achieve peace with your self-image.

The first thing that you must understand is the importance of uncovering the deceptive ideal—the one that celebrates society's distorted idea of a woman—and begin blessing the Godly attributes to which you aspire. You need to step into God's kingdom, where He is waiting to restore your self-image with peace and healing.

It is important to realize that this issue with your self-image is a much bigger conflict than you can handle on your own. To win, you must involve Father God in the battle. Walk this out in His kingdom (on earth as it is in heaven), where He is able to protect you from lies the enemy spreads. Begin to watch your conversation and listen for the words you speak concerning yourself and the bodies of others; become fully aware of the truth that what you say is what you get. You may think twice before declaring, "A moment on the lips, a lifetime on the hips."

Let's take a look at what Proverbs 18 says about the power of your words:

The words of a [discreet and wise] man's mouth are like deep waters [plenteous and difficult to fathom], and the fountain of skillful and godly wisdom is like a gushing stream [sparkling, fresh, pure, and life-giving].

To respect the person of the wicked and be partial to him, so as to deprive the [consistently] righteous of justice, is not good. A [self-confident] fool's lips bring contention, and his mouth invites a beating.

A [self-confident] fool's mouth is his ruin, and his lips are a snare to himself. The words of a whisperer or tail-bearer are as dainty morsels; they go down into the inner-most parts of the body.

A man's [moral] self shall be filled with the fruit of his mouth; and with the consequence of his words he must be satisfied [whether good or evil].

Death and life are in the power of the tongue, and they who indulge in it shall eat the fruit of it [for death or life].

Additionally, Matthew 12:37 states, "For by your words you will be justified *and* acquitted, and by your words you will be condemned *and* sentenced."

Confessing positive words over your body, as well as the bodies of others, is essential to achieving the very best *you*. Think about it: If you constantly gripe and complain about the attributes with which your Father God endowed you, what makes you think He will be willing to provide anything else for you to be ungrateful about? God cannot bless self-rejection and dishonor—it is not of Him.

When you begin to align your thoughts about your body image and weight with the Fruit of the Spirit, the supernatural grace of God begins to flow and serves as a foundation for Him to build upon. This foundation, the Fruits of the Spirit, includes love, joy, peace, patience, kindness, goodness, faithfulness, gentleness, and self-control (Galatians 5:22).

I realize that aspiring to this list is quite daunting, especially when you are dealing with your contrary flesh. A good place to begin is to ask yourself the following questions:

- Do I operate in the Fruits of the Spirit when it comes to my own self-image?
- Do I love myself and treat myself with respect and kindness?
- Have I displayed self-control and patience when it comes to my eating and exercise habits?
- Have I given it over to God, or am I operating out of my own self-will?
- Have I invited God into this area of my life?

The Fruits of the Spirit are of God; they originated with Him. When you allow God to meet you where you are, He is able to manifest His attributes within you. When you submit to His plan, God is always faithful and honors your decision; you will begin to witness His power transforming you from the inside out as you develop into the image He has of you.

Begin to lay hands on yourself, praying for and receiving the manifestation of the Fruits of the Spirit. Physically touch your body—specifically, the parts where you need healing. Thank God for the ability to be kind to yourself and to feel joy about the beautiful body He has given you. Honor God with this prayer:

Thank you, Lord, for blessing my beautiful arms, my hands, and my face. Thank you for my beautiful eyes and the perfect arch in my eyebrows. I thank You, God, for Your amazing creation. Thank you for my very life, Lord, because it is in You that I live and move and have my very being.

Touching yourself in this way, while admiring God's amazing creation, sparks a change in your heart because you are honoring God's workmanship. You are the most intimate manifestation of God's work on the earth. Praise Him for His goodness to you.

Soul Inceptions

Thoughts are powerful; your words can be the very weapon that hinders or halts your progress altogether.

Exalt the physical characteristics of others, especially those characteristics you aspire to obtain.

Begin to listen for words you speak over yourself—and the bodies of others—with full awareness that you receive what you speak.

Confessing positive words over your body, as well as the bodies of others, is essential in achieving your best physique.

Chapter 5

Reveal and Deal

For more than ten years, I have worked with thousands of women. Sadly, most of these women were so deeply filled with lies of failure that they couldn't even hear the advice I was sharing. By identifying with false messaging, they had based their self-worth on lies. They had defeated their weight loss plans before they even walked through my door.

Don't allow what you imagine that others may be thinking about you determine who you are, and definitely do not let past events identify you or your future. Base your identification on God, because through the blood of Jesus Christ, you are perfect to Him. When God lives in you, you become a recipient of His divine nature.

> *By means of these He has bestowed on us His precious and exceedingly great promises, so that through them that you may escape [by flight] from the moral decay [rottenness and corruption] that is in the world because of covetousness [lust and greed], and become sharers [partakers] of the divine nature.*
>
> 2 Peter 1:4

Remember, Satan is a master of manipulation, and he loves to speak lies into your consciousness. Don't trust what he says! Instead, rely on the unwavering truth of God's word.

As I've shared, I married at the age of twenty-four and gave birth to my daughter fifteen months later. During the pregnancy, my now ex-husband became involved with someone else, and I was divorced before Olivia was five months old. These circumstances, occurring when I was already in a vulnerable state, were a severe blow to my self-esteem.

As a result of these overwhelming events, Satan had intentionally planted a poisonous weed in my subconsciousness. With its growth came feelings of self-doubt, mistrust, and a never-ending mental parade of "If I had only …" thoughts. *If I had only been a better wife. If I had only been more attractive. If I had only gained less weight with the pregnancy.*

Do you realize that God is faithful and will bless the broken road you find yourself traveling on—when you are willing to offer up your broken heart to Him? I don't want to imply that this is an easy process, because you will have some revealing and dealing to do. You may carry so much heaviness within your heart that you are being eaten alive—literally. Someone may have given up on you or purposely wounded you; it could be your mother, father, husband, boyfriend, sister, brother, friend, or even a stranger. And you now measure your self-worth by that incident. If you want to change course toward a new future, you must identify and reveal the weed-infested, contaminated ideas that are growing within your consciousness.

I have heard it said that the only thing a seed knows is that it needs to grow. This is true, no matter what type of seed or where it is sown. It doesn't matter if it is a daisy seed or a dandelion seed. Under favorable conditions, any seed will grow. And contrary to what you might think, not all seeds were created to be sown into the ground. Some seeds are designed specifically to be sown into your mind and others into your spirit. Your soul possesses the seeds of thought, and you also have the ability to sow ideas, attitudes, and prejudices into another person.

Once a thought seed is rooted in your mind, it grows into an emotion and then flowers into a belief. A belief then manifests itself through your body by producing an action. When seeds of negativity are sown, the end result is a garden full of physical and mental disease. But you can have confidence that, just as in the Gospel of Matthew, Jesus's promise of healing remains true today if you steadfastly believe that He will honor His word.

> *Then He touched their eyes, saying, "According to your faith and trust and reliance [on the power invested in me] be it done to you." And their eyes were opened.*
>
> Matthew 9:29–30

Throughout my career, the majority of the women I have counseled had been prescribed more than two types of medications to control depression, blood pressure, cholesterol, or other ailments. While working as a personal trainer, I discovered that many of my clients were desperately trying to find ways to superglue the pieces of their broken hearts back together. Often they were suffering from an abundance of weeds that had been sown into their subconscious minds. As they confided in me, I began to notice a direct correlation between the toxic weeds of a client's beliefs and the status of her weight and health.

I remember one particular conversation with a woman who recounted a painful period that had occurred during her childhood. She recalled that her parent had asked her why she was not thin like other children. While she was only ten years old, she was put on very strict dieting regimens. However, what was even more damaging to her self-esteem was overhearing her parents discussing her weight with relatives.

I had several clients who, as young adults, had dreaded that Saturday trip to their grandparents' house. Inevitably, the first remark they heard upon arrival would be a comment regarding how much weight they had gained or lost. And, if a young woman was really lucky, old family videos would be played so that the family could show her date how chunky she had been during puberty. The accompanying soundtrack generally included, "You know, she didn't always look like she does today." And then everyone would have a good laugh at my client's expense.

I once heard the mother of a very dear friend of mine greet him with the words, "Oh wow! You look fat!" Yet he was not overweight by any scientific or social standard. At the dinner table, when dessert was served, my friend's mother made it a point to tell him (in front of the entire dinner party) that he should not have any dessert. While my client's plate remained empty, his mother and the other guests proceeded to eat strawberry swirled cheesecake in front of him.

Another client was a sweet young woman whose parents had divorced. When her father remarried and began to have children with his new wife, he told my client that he would no longer be responsible for her, as he needed to provide for his new family. The emotions that took root from that experience were abandonment, confusion, and rejection.

It's well known that, as children, most of us strive to make our parents proud. When intentional seeds of outright rejection are sown by a parent or other adult family member, beliefs such as "I am replaceable," and "I will never let anyone get close enough to hurt me like that again," can grow quite rapidly and be very destructive.

With time, the father's seeds of rejection led to dysfunctional actions. My client began isolating herself after her parents' divorce, and, year after year, she continued to steadily gain weight. Subconsciously, she used her weight as a defense mechanism to excuse herself from social activities and avoid opportunities to get to know others. She justified her behavior with the belief that, because of her weight, people wouldn't like her much anyway. This dysfunctional behavior kept her confined within her body, which eventually weighed more than three hundred pounds.

These are disturbing examples of how our layered beliefs are formed about food. Once these beliefs take control, we begin to subconsciously apply them to future comments, ideas, and experiences. Extreme examples of intentionally sowing weeds in others include sexual and physical abuse. Clients who have been victimized in this way often feel protected by the additional weight they carry. The beliefs that sprouted in their consciousness as a result of the abuse were confirmed: "If I am unattractive, no one will harm me." These women allowed the effects of rape and other sexually perverted tragedies to keep them from achieving God's desire for their physical body. Even if they attempted to regain a healthy body, in many cases a sensual glance from a stranger was all it took to cause their progress to come to a screeching halt.

God desires for you to recognize His image in yourself. To do this, you must be willing to redefine beauty. You were created in God's image, and He delights in you. He longs to see you embrace a new image—an image that would have existed before the sexually perverted tragedy created an interruption in the natural order of your life. Let go of the belief that you are protected by added weight, and reject the lie that you are in some way responsible for the situation that occurred.

Recognize that you have been inappropriately punishing yourself by withdrawing from the nutrients you so desperately need. The enemy has imprisoned you within your body by encouraging you to believe that your mission is to become unattractive at all costs, even if it means disfiguring yourself. Using terror and torment, Satan has convinced you that the rape (or other tragedy) can occur again at any given moment. He whispers that you are ultimately responsible for what has happened—and what could happen again—and that your beauty is a curse. These are lies from the very pit of hell. With a Godly determination, you need to overcome the power and effects of rape (or any other sexually perverted tragedy) and no longer allow them to hold you back from developing into the person God designed you to become.

Inherently, the fear of recurrence results in a fear of beginning, a state of decline, or a plateau in your progress. The promise in the book of Joshua gives confidence that as children of God, no one will be able to stand against you and that God will remain with you always. He will never leave you or forsake you. You can boldly declare that "my enemies stumble and fall before they can reach me" (Joshua 1:5, Psalm 27:2). As a child of God, you have access to the spiritual weapons listed in His word, and you can use them to combat a repeated onset of this type of mental torment. You are covered and protected in the name of Jesus. "Fear not. I am with you," says the Lord (Psalm 41:10). Don't ever let a fear of recurrence keep you from claiming all God has prepared for your future.

It is time to redefine beauty. Right now, I want you to jot down on a piece of paper at least ten words that describe your physical characteristics and attributes.

Ready? Go!

Now that you've completed a list that describes you, on another piece of paper write ten words that describe Christ.

Go ahead, I'll wait.

Compare your lists. Do any of the characteristics appear on both pieces of paper? I certainly hope so! Are you able to see yourself through your Father's eyes? You should; He made you in His image.

The harsh reality is that, too often, the weeds of your past encroach into the files of your consciousness. This chapter is not written to point fingers and place blame, as that would do nothing but paralyze you within the role of a victim. Continuing to identify yourself as a victim prohibits change from occurring in your life. The fact is that you, alone, are responsible for what is growing in the garden of your consciousness. You cannot blame your condition on the actions of others. While someone else may have planted a weed, the choice of whether to continue watering and nurturing a weed or to pull it out is yours to make.

Awareness is the key; there is power that comes with being made aware of your rights, your responsibilities, and your authority. Victory resides within the truth that you have the authority to uproot weeds, sow a new crop, and reap a healthy bountiful harvest.

I encourage you to take a few moments to think back over your life. On the following pages, write down the intentional actions of others that have planted weeds that have affected your life.

Workbook

Weed of Thought / Experience / Translation:

Example: Betrayal from a loved one / adultery / forsaking of marital vows

Rooted Emotion

Example: Dishonored, rejected, cheap

Bloomed Belief

Example: I am inadequate and must compensate for that. I can no longer trust men. I am independent.

Inherited Action of Dysfunction

Example: I attempt to control my environment to the point of extremity through Anorexia Nervosa.

Your Turn:

1. Weed of Thought / Experience / Translation:

    Rooted Emotion:

    Bloomed Belief:

    Inherited Action:

2. Weed of Thought / Experience / Translation:

    Rooted Emotion:

    Bloomed Belief:

    Inherited Action:

> *For he who sows to his own flesh [lower nature, sensuality], will from the flesh reap decay and ruin and destruction. But he who sows to the Spirit, will [from the Spirit] reap eternal life.*
>
> Galatians 6:8

There is one additional area I want to address. The seeds you sow into your impressionable children—whether intentionally or unintentionally—can determine how they will view, think about, and care for their own bodies. As a parent, you need to be aware that a quick trip to the dressing room to try on a pair of jeans can make a dramatic impact on the life of your five-year-old daughter. Standing in front of the three-way mirror to get a better look at your bottom half, she watches as you mumble words of disapproval, pinch at your thighs, and try to suck in your gut. Behaving this way in front your child may not be the best idea.

Instead, when your child is with you, you should compliment your attributes as you look in the mirror. Don't look for flaws. Instead, positively affirm that you are a beautiful, sexy woman of God. It is important to feel that you deserve the victory in this battle for your self-esteem, to model healthy behavior, and to encourage it in your sons and daughters.

Additionally, it is vital that you speak positive words over your children and create positive plans for them. If they are making unwise decisions, don't speak condemnation into their lives; this will only allow a rooted emotion to take hold. Instead, pray for your children and allow the Fruits of the Spirit to govern your response. Through your actions and attitude, guide your children toward positive behavior. Trust the Holy Spirit to speak to them and work God's will through them.

I've heard it said, "You create your world with your words, and the only one who gives anything its meaning is you." Since you cannot control the meaning your children (or anyone, for that matter) will give to your words, you must strive to use words of kindness, goodness, strength, and power, and make them your reality. Remember, what you focus on expands in your life.

Soul Inceptions

When negative words and images are implanted in our minds, the end result is a heart and soul full of manifested disease, both physical and mental.

*You cannot be responsible, nor can you control, what others speak into your life. However, you **are** responsible for the negativisms broadcasting in your consciousness.*

The choice to nurture the negative thoughts and images others have spoken into your life is your very own.

Your spirit has the authority to annihilate, excavate, and weed out intruding rejections.

Chapter 6

Self-Destructive Behavior: The Silent Sower

I want to expose another type of contaminated weed that is, most often, sown unintentionally. I call these self-destructive weeds. I have come to the realization that self-destruction can be a learned behavior that is passed down from generation to generation, and it reveals itself in many forms.

My self-destruction developed as a result of watching my mother pass away with lung cancer. Although she had smoked from a very young age, watching her suffer with that disease caused self-destructive thoughts to seep into my subconscious mind. I began to believe that the only way I could maintain a connection with my mother was by repeating the pattern of suffering she had endured. Why did I buy into this? *Because I had learned self-destructive behavior.* Although I did not smoke—in fact, I was a crusader for health for the very reason that smoking had killed my mother—I attempted to destroy myself in another way: by withholding food and nutrients and taking every diet pill available. I may not have been smoking, but my actions caused great stress and destruction to my body.

For a period of time, the familiarity of the self-destructive process allowed me to comfortably blame, punish, and eventually wrap myself up in the chains of regret for everything I could have or should have done differently. The *should-haves* and *could-haves* consumed me with guilt for every failed situation: when my mother was sick, when my brother took his life, when my marriage failed, when I made mistakes as a mother.

The seed sown in this case was that of my mother's self-destructive behavior of smoking. Unintentionally, I allowed self-destruction to play a large part in my life. As I compulsively chased perfection, the seeds of self-destruction became rooted in my subconscious and led me toward negligence and a lack of responsibility toward my physical body. The fully grown belief bloomed into feelings of unworthiness, and I continued in my own self-destructive cycle.

The nature of a weed is to grow aggressively, even under adverse circumstances, even without proper nutrients or watering. (It takes very little effort to keep weeds thriving in your yard or in your mind.) The rapid growth of a weed pushes out and chokes desirable vegetation—your healthy, fruit-bearing beliefs—depleting them of the energy and strength they need to grow and preventing you from escaping the toxic belief that started the entire process.

Just as the tiny parachute of a dandelion seed is dislodged, rides along with the wind, and is easily sown in a new location, the entire self-destructive cycle can be replicated with very little effort. This process is the work of Satan attempting to inhibit the growth of desirable fruit and attempting to destroy you from the inside out. (The enemy loves nothing more than to initiate and then cultivate our destruction.) The good news is that you have a secret weapon: you were made in the likeness of God.

> *So God created man in his own image, in the image and likeness of God He created him; male and female he created them.*
> Genesis 1:27

It would have been nearly effortless, despite the potentially devastating consequences, for me to continue living a life of self-destruction, completing yet another cycle in this vicious pattern of suffering—and passing it on to the next generation. Fortunately, the Lord intervened on my behalf (and on behalf of my daughter). He dealt with me in this area by making me aware of my actions and revealing the consequences of my behavior.

It is imperative to take authority over your health and over your body. Using the gifts of the kingdom, begin breaking the yokes of your inherited curses.

> *I call heaven and earth to witness this day against you that I have set before you life and death, the blessings and the curses; therefore choose life, that you and your descendants may live and may love the Lord your God, obey his voice, and cling to Him. For he is your life and the length of your days that you may dwell in the land which the Lord swore to give to your fathers, to Abraham, Isaac, and Jacob.*
>
> Deuteronomy 30: 19–20

You must fight to fulfill God's calling for your life. I can guarantee that you were not created to live a dreadful life and then dig your way into an early grave. You do not have to be a victim of your circumstances; you not a prisoner of your genes or your jeans. You have the capability and responsibility to recognize and break the cycle of self-destructive behaviors, including drug use, alcoholism, smoking, obesity, bulimia, anorexia, and other eating disorders. The risks associated with these behaviors are well-documented and include coronary heart disease, hypertension, stroke, diabetes, increased risks for various cancers, osteoarthritis, and depression. You owe it to the next generation to bind these destructive behaviors and cast them out in the name of Jesus! It is your responsibility to break the cycle.

> *For though we walk [live] in the flesh, we are not carrying on our warfare according to the flesh and using mere human weapons. For the weapons of our warfare are not physical [weapons of flesh and blood], but they are mighty before God for the overthrow and destruction of strongholds.*
>
> 2 Corinthians 10:3–4

You are history in the making. The time has come to openly declare your heart's desires to the Father. He wants to free you from the devouring and captivity Satan has placed on your body. When you partner with God, He will break the curses your family has suffered and provide liberty for you and all generations who come after you.

There were days when I felt so hopeless that I was unable to reign in my self-destructive addictions. Fortunately, it didn't matter how I felt, because Jesus had a firm hold on me, and He has a hold on you as well. I had nothing to gain by continuing to surrender my life to prescription diet pills and the tormenting demonic force of starvation. Like me, you have nothing to gain by remaining absorbed with your own destructive vices.

Be honest with yourself. Are you committed and willing to move forward in Christ or do your fear-based excuses continually hold you back? Let them go—fear is the most dangerous mindset of all. There is no benefit to holding on to emotional garbage that will eventually manifest itself as physical garbage. Spiritual constipation sets in when you remain more comfortable with your current set of circumstances—regardless of how poisonous they have become—rather than risk exploring where God wants to lead you.

You have been exposed to abandonment, shame, and disappointment through human experiences, and these interactions have left you questioning your self-worth. The truth is that your experiences do not identify who you are. God is in charge of the identification department. He is the greatest lover of your life and delights in your complete fulfillment. God never disappoints. Drop your guard, let go of the comfortable, and let Him take control.

Take the next few moments to recognize the unintentional sowing of self-destructive behaviors in your life and where they may have originated. Use the following guide to help you expose weeds, emotions, beliefs, and dysfunctional behaviors. I also invite you to use this time to list any self-destructive behavior you may have acquired as a result.

Workbook

Weed of Thought Experience Translation

Example: Watching my mother choose to smoke and observing her death and the circumstances that came thereafter

Rooted Emotions

Example: Fearful, perfectionist, self-condemning, and self-obsessed

Bloomed Belief

Example: I am undeserving of life

Inherited Action of Dysfunction

Example: Drug addiction, Anorexia Nervosa

Your Turn:

1. Weed of Thought Experience Translation:

    Rooted Emotions:

    Bloomed Belief:

    Inherited Action:

2. Weed of Thought Experience Translation:

   Rooted Emotions:

   Bloomed Belief:

   Inherited Action:

Soul Inceptions

Self-destruction can be a learned behavior passed down generationally.

Although self-destructive behavior can externalize into its original form, unusual behaviors can, regrettably, emerge.

It takes very little effort to breed self-destruction.

Chapter 7

Weeding Out Your Soul with Forgiveness

Once you have identified your own "weeds," the question then becomes, "What should you do with the weeds that have been sown deep within the files of your subconscious?"

When your files become filled to capacity and begin to burst, what action do you take? Do you just create another file to accommodate the toxic weeds headed your way? Are you going to continue pressing "open" and "replay" in your mental computer? Or are you willing to hit "delete"?

If you want to know how to delete the subconscious file that contains the destructive weeds, the answer is *forgiveness!*

So [instead of further rebuke, now] you should rather turn and [graciously] forgive and comfort and encourage [your brother], to keep him from being overwhelmed by obsessive sorrow and despair.

I therefore beg you to reinstate him in your affections and assure him of your love for him; For this was my purpose in writing you, to test your attitude and to see if you would stand the test; whether you are obedient and altogether agreeable [to following of my orders] in everything.

If you forgive anyone anything, I too forgive that one; and what I have forgiven, if I have forgiven anything, has been for your sakes in the presence [and with the approval] of Christ [the Messiah], To keep Satan from getting the advantage over us; for we are not ignorant of his wiles, and intentions.

2 Corinthians 2:7–11

The person who caused your offense may very well be incapable of comprehending, or oblivious to, the pain he or she has created. Or, that person might suffer from remorse and be waiting for your forgiveness, while you're still tightly gripping the offense. Holding onto an offense has the power to destroy you from the inside out. Do you want sweet and lasting freedom? Forgive, forgive, and forgive!

I realize how painful the act of forgiving can be, but it is essential to your complete renovation. When your act of acquittal toward the offender puts an end to the blame, you are no longer held hostage to the situation. The struggle you encounter with acquitting your offender arises when you believe that there are certain individuals who do not deserve the mercy of forgiveness.

Bitterness had made itself at home in my heart since my husband's affair, and my attitude toward men—all men—had become downright nasty. This kind of hatred is dangerous and stimulates risky conduct. Men became nothing more than a warm body on a cold and lonely night; to me, that's all they were good for as I became determined that I could—and would—take care of everything else I needed. Unfortunately, my ugly disposition led to a few much-regretted one-night stands.

Truly forgiving my former husband and his lover was the catalyst that allowed my healing to take place. Forgiveness caused my bleeding heart to miraculously be sutured. My choice to forgive immediately unleashed my soul from a state of restless doubt, suspicion, and shame.

My breakthrough occurred when I humbly realized that, as a sinner, I didn't deserve the gift of God's forgiveness any more than those who had hurt me deserved it. All of us have been freely extended the very same mercy from a loving and compassionate God. Forgiveness uncorked a flood of benefits in my life, restored my ability to love, and gave God the opportunity to introduce my soul mate.

When I asked God how I would ever again be able to trust men again, He replied, *"My love, it is not the man you need to trust, it is I."* Even while I was still incapable of placing my confidence in men, Jesus only asked that I trust Him with the men in my life. In order for healing to take place, however, my actions needed to demonstrate that I trusted God, so I began to handle my body honorably. That meant that I needed to forgive myself first.

With God's help, I left behind the woman I used to be—the one who was addicted to perfection, involved in self-destructive behavior, living with shame and regret, and afraid to trust—and I have never been the same again. I now shamelessly walk hand in hand with God. I have placed all my trust and hopes in the Lord, and He has been a loving and faithful companion.

The relationship I now share with my former husband, as well as with my former in-laws, is healthy and whole. God has provided wonderful grandparents for my daughter. None of this would have been possible without my choosing to forgive. I could have held onto the offense—after all, this was my choice—and in the process, I would have robbed my daughter and myself of the wonderful relationships we enjoy today. You may be wondering what happened to all the trauma I suffered. Well, God delivered me from that through his promise in Jeremiah, where He revealed that His plan for me was life, not death.

> *For I know the thoughts and plans that I have for you, says the Lord, thoughts and plans for welfare and peace and not for evil, to give you hope in your final outcome.*
>
> Jeremiah 29:11

It took some time, but I finally realized that God was not to blame for all the hardship I had experienced in my life. I learned that, much like the situation portrayed in *Star Wars*, there is a dark side in this world intent on destruction, and Satan (and all of hell) is very real.

Jesus was sent to earth to die so that anyone who calls on His name could obtain legal immunity from the consequences of hell on earth. He desires for you to experience heaven on earth as you walk free from Satan's plan of destruction. As 2 Corinthians 5:17 reveals, anyone who asks will become a new creation in Christ and the old person will no longer exist. As Jesus presents this amazing opportunity for you to transform your life, you have an obligation to extend a brand-new beginning to the person responsible for hurting you.

Also in 2 Corinthians, the Bible states that we are to forgive for the sake of the offender as well as for the sake of ourselves—with Christ in mind as He forgave us. Forgiveness frees both you and your offender from the bondage of emotional chaos and crushes the plot of Satan who desires only to kill, steal, and destroy.

Ready to start forgiving? My suggestion is to find a quiet place where you will have at least thirty minutes to yourself. (This is a good exercise for right before you lie down to sleep at night.) Visualize a calm place. It may be a beautiful, empty beach filled with sunlight, pink sand, and a sea breeze. Or you may prefer to visualize yourself sitting near a fireplace, in a comfortable Victorian chair, with a warm cup of tea. The surroundings you choose aren't critical; envision any serene place.

In your calm and peaceful setting, meet with each person who has filled your weed-infested files. Invite Jesus to sit between you and the individual who has caused you pain. Refer to the lists you have created in the previous chapters. Repeat the following prayer as many times as needed until you have met with and prayed for every person who has given offense.

Heavenly Father:
I forgive the person sitting before me now. I pray that he [or she] will no longer be overwhelmed by excessive sorrow. I recognize the weed of action sown into my life by this person, and I relinquish blame, releasing it in Your holy name.

Lord, lead me to the garden of my subconsciousness as together we abolish the emotions that have taken root by tilling, pulling, and annihilating the negative bloomed belief. I forgive myself and accept freedom from shame and guilt as I acknowledge that You have died for my sins and forgiven me, paying the price for my salvation.

Based on Your covenant, I bind and cast out self-destructive behavior, as it has no legal standing over me. I take cover under Your protection. I rebuke and purge myself of all self-destructive behaviors, realizing that the authority You have given me forces them to completely halt their influence over me.

Jesus, I now open the door to receive new, healthy growth. Flood the gardens of my mind with peace and love; restore my body and physical well-being. I pray in Your name. Amen.

This exercise has done wonders in softening my heart, as well as helping me gain a better understanding of the individuals who have polluted the files of my subconscious garden.

Soul Inceptions

Forgiveness is essential to your complete remaking.

Regarding your enemy: When your act of acquittal puts an end to blame, you are no longer hostage to that situation or experience.

Forgiveness uncorks a flood of God-given benefits.

Chapter 8

Vital Vision

Create a true, vital, active, healthy image of your body. If it is difficult for you to do this, keep in mind that the hairs on your head were numbered and you were made in the very likeness of God. You were intelligently designed and predetermined with great care and consideration.

> *But [even] the very hairs of your head are all numbered. Do not be struck with fear or seized with alarm; you are of greater worth than many [flocks] of sparrows.*
>
> Luke 12:7

Your body is a sacred gift from the Father and should be treated with as much respect as you afford any other gift He has placed in your life. As a woman, you no doubt go to great lengths to nourish and care for your relationships, spouses, and children. You need to invest the same devotion and commitment in caring for yourself.

Your body is your greatest ally, your oldest friend and, most importantly, the vehicle for your soul and spirit. You require a strong body and clear mind to carry out all the wonderful plans God has in store for you. And you better believe God wants you to take authority—using the gifts of His kingdom—to become the thriving, strong, beautiful woman He designed you to be.

Ask God to impart His vision of you *to* you. You will begin to see beautiful pictures of yourself interacting with a soul mate yet unmet (or your spouse), and perhaps even your children or unborn children, grandchildren, and even great-grandchildren. You will see yourself sharing the Word of God with people you have yet to meet as you come to the realization that you have a sacred responsibility to fulfill: creating a healthy future for lives, memories, and experiences. God has bestowed upon each of us many talents. You may have a gift of wisdom, speaking, healing, writing, loving, creating, ministering, or mentoring—all of which require you to act responsibly toward your body and your gift.

Instead of marveling at the person God has created and the future He has planned for you, too often you remain captive in your body, fighting the weight loss (or weight gain) battle day after day. The enemy robs you of God's vision. You focus on what the scale reveals in the morning, struggle to get beyond a number that overshadows your entire day, and, ultimately, your obsession with that number derails God's plan for you.

I, for one, do not wish to stand before the Lord on the day I arrive in heaven and have Him say,

Angela, I created you with beautiful gifts. Why didn't you use them? Why did you squander them? I have always been there with you, just as I am before you today. My strength was yours for the taking; all you had to do was reach out and take it. Why wouldn't you receive it? Although there were many who gave up on you, I always believed in you. Why did you choose to give up on yourself?

You need to realize that the Holy Spirit has no limit on the amount of energy, power, and strength He will make available when you are utilizing that energy for God's glory, will, and purpose. His grace, power, and healing are yours for the taking. It's your move. Are you willing to accept what God has offered?

It is not God's will (or judgment or punishment) to watch you struggle with high blood pressure, high cholesterol, weight issues, body image, or any other affliction. You, however, must be the one who decides to exercise your faith and walk in God's supernatural strength. Simply put, your faith without corresponding actions is dead. While Jesus wants to gift you with the supernatural, receiving it requires action on your part. Even Peter had to get out of the boat to demonstrate that God had given him the ability to walk on water.

In the midst of my recovery, the Holy Spirit provided me with a non-negotiable confirmation regarding the dimensions and proportions of my body. Relying on God's intended design for me meant that I needed to respond by throwing out the scale. Since I had been bound by numbers for years, taking this action was an important step of obedience in creating a healthy vision.

If you ask God to reveal His blueprint of your body (your form, shape, size, and makeup), without a doubt, He will provide you with an image of the genuine you He created. Humbly submit yourself to His vision and come into agreement with your Creator concerning the dimensions of your body. Once you hear from Him, a comforting quietness will settle within the depths of your heart. Be sure to write down God's word as a reminder of what He has planned for you. If you're willing to accept it, His promise will become an unalterable contract between you and your Father.

And in the event that you are planning on negotiating with God, I am living proof, here to tell you it won't work. God's word is His final authority. If you engage in a conversation with Him, God will make it very clear how much you are meant to eat, what you are meant to eat, and how much you are meant to exercise. There is no compromise when it comes to God's instruction to you.

You have the ability to listen to your body and know when you are satisfied. You are capable of making good food choices and winning the battle with your weight. Success is an accumulation of one good decision after another that produces the desired results. You make progress one meal at a time.

And whatever you ask for in prayer, having faith and [really] believing, you will receive.

Matthew 21:22

Soul Inceptions

Your body is a sacred gift from the Father.

Your body is your greatest ally, your oldest friend, and, most importantly, the vehicle of your soul and spirit.

You require an able-bodied vehicle to carry out God's purpose for your life.

Come into a mutual agreement with your Creator concerning the size of your body.

Chapter 9

Reevaluating Fixations

If it is impossible to measure the greatness of God on a scale, how can you measure the man or woman He created on one? If you can't fit God into a pill bottle, why do you think you are going to find solutions in one? You must let go of the assumption that you will find your answer in food—or the lack thereof. Turn away from the lie that food, weight loss pills, or the number on the scale is the final authority that will dictate your future.

There are many great health and fitness tools available and a seemingly unending supply of information to be absorbed. However, if you are not inviting God into your situation, you can read all the books, attend all the seminars, and even hire a personal trainer and you will still miss the gift of transformation and freedom. What I am saying is this: don't place your trust in earthly tools and knowledge alone, specifically when it pertains to your weight. It is critical that you find a proper spiritual balance in the midst of all the chaos. Allow the tools to be just that—tools. Realize that they cannot provide the solutions you are seeking; you will only find answers through your faith in God. The tools can assist as you begin to make weight and body image changes, but only the Spirit of God can sustain those changes and give you the ability to break bonds and habits that have created your current circumstances.

The Holy Spirit will provide you with the strength that will empower you to make consistently healthy choices and create good habits that will last throughout your lifetime. When you trust in God, an awesome grace flows into your life. As I turned away from trying to do it my way and entered into covenant with God, I lost the desire for those things that were harmful for me. As you let God take control of your situation and learn to rely on Him, you'll find that midnight burger and ice cream, that cigarette, that diet pill, or the idea of skipping another meal will become less and less desirable.

While exercise is a critical part of your healthy lifestyle, it's not the entire answer. More than 80 percent of your health results come from the choices you make about food.[1] The greatest strides you will make in the area of your health will be outside of the gym or your workout.

Zechariah 4:6 states that it is "Not by might, nor by power, but by my spirit says the lord of hosts." As a matter of fact, whenever you attempt to *will* something to happen and try to force it, the result is generally a dead end. Remember, you achieve success not by *your* strength, but through *His* strength in you. What a relief it is to realize you don't need to depend on your own will power; it is God's power of will in you that causes you to triumph. You are not alone in this journey.

I quickly learned that my self-righteous will was not capable of restoring my body to its intended weight. It was exhilarating when I began to operate in the revelation that I could rely on the Holy Spirit to guide my choices regarding what foods to eat, how much to eat, and how often I should eat. I simply paused and prayed before I put anything in my mouth, then I waited for God's peace and discernment. It is so important to take the time to listen! Too often, we are quick to dismiss a message from the Holy Spirit as nonsense. Act in haste at your own peril.

A few years ago, I attended a festival sponsored by my husband's company. Before the evening of the big banquet, I decided to catch up with some old friends over lunch. As I sat down to enjoy sushi, I distinctly heard a voice—one that sounded much like my own—say, *This fish is no good.* I quickly disregarded the caution as a random thought running through my mind, and I proceeded to enjoy a nice meal. Sure enough, later that evening I began to suffer with symptoms of food poisoning.

When you are committed to listening for the voice of the Holy Spirit, you become completely moldable by the work of God's hands. When you allow Him, He will guide your actions, help you avoid disaster, and steer you to success.

During my recovery God requested that I rid my life of my scale and every other earthly weight loss fixation I had accumulated. Among other things, I tossed out fad diet books, diet pills, diet food, and calorie counters. I was asked to take my focus and the energy I was putting into that dysfunctional lifestyle and invest them in my relationship with God. He desired that I put more trust in Him than I did in my scale.

As a result of this process, I discovered that focusing on the numbers is much like having a noose wrapped around your neck. While you are making a desperate attempt to remove the rope, it becomes tighter and tighter. If you attempt to pull it off by your own strength, you end up choking yourself and wondering why those numbers on the scale are going in the wrong direction. Instead, step back, take a deep breath, and realize that achieving a healthy wieght is not accomplished by your might or power. Then, loosen the noose at the base with full confidence that you can do all things through God, who will give you the strength.

The moment I set my focus on God, a feeling of peace encompassed me, and anxieties about my issues with weight and food began to disappear. I was no longer engaged in a struggle between wrong food versus right food, the *can* and *can't* haves, or bacon versus bananas. My unnatural drive for perfectionism began to diminish, and my soul became quiet. I found myself in transition—in new and unknown territory—and I could see myself for what I had become: exhausted and unpleasant.

Without the comfortable (but unhealthy) rigidity of operating in my own will, I became miserably aware of how void I had become.

I realized that I had been putting all my effort into my outward appearance while ignoring what was taking place on the inside. I had been so consumed with my own disturbed anguish that I had nothing comforting or pleasant to offer anyone else. I had become miserable, and I made all who were around me feel distressed—especially those who were willing to dine with me. Before I could see what I had become, I had to place my focus completely on God. When I began to compare myself with His perfect standard, I was shocked by the disparity.

You will guard him and keep him in perfect and constant peace whose mind [both its inclination and its character] is stayed on You, because he commits himself to You, leans on You, and hopes confidently in You.

Isaiah 26:3

An interesting fact in the world of nutrition states that eating food with guilt and stress causes forms of emotional toxicity[2] to be created. This toxicity negatively manipulates a healthy metabolic function and results in increasing percentages of body fat.[3] When you set your focus on Father God, rather than your food, you have taken an important first step in the process of becoming a healthier person. The ultimate goal is to present your body with the highest quality, nutrient-enriched foods available, and make Godly choices about what you introduce into your body.

Soul Inceptions

Let go of the fact that the weight loss pill or the number on the scale is the final authority that dictates your outcome.

The more you seek God and rely on Him, the less you will desire those foods that are not good for you.

Before you put anything in your mouth, slow down, pray, and wait for peace and discernment.

Chapter 10

Fueling the Vehicle of Your Soul

As I shared earlier, your body is the vehicle of your soul and spirit. So I have to ask, "What type of fuel do you put in your engine: unleaded, super unleaded, or premium?" When you are fixated on the opinions of this world, your spirit is contaminated with dirty fuel, and your body is poisoned with toxins, it becomes very difficult to hear the voice of the Holy Spirit.

Clean fuel is critical to strong performance and long engine life; fuel injectors have tiny openings that clog easily with even small amounts of debris. While the fuel filter (your liver) does a good job of filtering fuel, it is not perfect. Over time deposits of fat, dirt, and tiny particles (toxins) lodge themselves in the injectors, clogging your arteries. These pollutants can clog the injectors and prevent them from delivering the fuel the engine, your heart, needs. If these conditions are not addressed, over time your car (body) will begin to feel sluggish and sometimes refuse to run properly. How can you accomplish what God has called you to do when it is a struggle to get out of bed because your system is overwhelmed with fat, dirt, and toxins?

The soil where our food is grown and the air we breathe are loaded with chemicals, pesticides, and petrochemicals that did not exist during biblical times. Factory-made processed foods with unidentified food additives are commonplace in our grocery stores and on our pantry shelves. Our meats are routinely injected with antibiotics and hormones. Nutritional experts have labeled flour, sugar, and salt the three white devils because they are highly addictive and habit-forming, yet they have no nutritional value and are not efficiently processed by the body. The book of Ezekiel reveals that during ancient times, breads and cakes did not contain these ingredients. Instead, commonly used ingredients were amaranth, barley, beans, lentils, millet, and spelt.

In my opinion, many of the synthesized foods being processed today are not in the best health interests of the consumer. I encourage you to begin investigating the inexpensive chemicals the United States Food and Drug Administration (FDA) is approving for inclusion in your foods. These chemicals are popular with food manufacturers because they permit low production costs and extremely high profit margins. Furthermore, these chemicals contain addictive non-nutritional agents which leave you hungry, prompting you to purchase and consume ever-larger quantities of processed foods.

I believe there are many objectionable actions taking place within the food production industry that have not yet been revealed to the public. I believe there may also be widespread deception that needs to be exposed so that consumers can make informed decisions to avoid the toxic buildup that results from consuming dangerous ingredients and additives. The most common symptoms of toxic buildup in your body include emotional stress, constipation, sluggishness or low energy, lack of motivation, strong food cravings, high sugar consumption, caffeine dependency, and unidentifiable lingering illness.

You should pray over your food for protection from toxins and unhealthy ingredients. You can also go one step further—take authority over what you put into your tank; elect to make less-toxic choices. These types of actions are important steps to maintaining strength in your body and clarity in your mind.

Tina the Toxin: A Parable

Tina has just started a fabulous new diet. To achieve her weight-loss goal, all she needs to do is eat only cabbage soup and bacon. Excitedly, she begins the first day of her new eating regime: bacon for breakfast, cabbage soup for lunch, cabbage soup for snack, cabbage soup for dinner ... and then, BAM! Her head begins to pound. Tina is exhausted, agitated, and becomes quite unpleasant to be around. As the kids begin pestering her about their dinner, she whips together some macaroni and cheese. The food begins to entice her. The aroma is almost more than she can bear and, as it beckons her, she begins to snarl back at it.

She grudgingly serves the children dinner as her husband walks through the door—late again. You better believe that if he is having dinner tonight, he will be eating leftover cabbage soup, and that's about *all* he is going to have for the remainder of the evening (if you know what I mean).

The night spirals into complete chaos as the family caps their busy day with an unsatisfying and unhealthy meal. After the children finally fall asleep, a desperately hungry Tina recalls the box of Hostess Ding Dongs in the pantry. They tempt her, and she succumbs to the moist chocolate cake and creamy vanilla frosting. It has been a stressful day, she rationalizes, and she deserves a treat. Somewhere between her fourth and fifth cupcake, her guilt sets in. Tina turns to her husband and sarcastically thanks him for placing the Ding Dongs in the grocery cart last week. Feeling poorly about herself and her choices, Tina initiates an argument. Unfortunately, the evening ends with hostility and frustration.

Reading this parable, I'm sure you realize the behavior that Tina exhibited is not of God. Yet, all too frequently many of us fall into similar traps set by the food choices we make.

Today, why not take time to reevaluate your thoughts and words so they align with your intentional purpose to reclaim your healthy body. Resolve to be free from words like *diet* and associated terms that allude to deprivation. Let's face it, the words "lose" and "loss" rarely bring good associations to mind. *Cheating* insinuates an urge to victimize or defraud and, within the context of dieting, most often *you* are that victim who is being harmed. Refrain from becoming involved with anything that might so easily lead you to become a double-crosser and that associates itself with lustfulness. After all, when you go on a diet—any type of diet—you are willfully taking matters into your own hands. When you lust after a desired physical appearance apart from God, you hinder Him from creating the future He has planned for you.

Realize that sometimes you are more defiled by what comes out of your mouth than by what goes in your body. (See Matthew 15:11.) You are no longer "starting again on Monday," because from this point forward, you are always "on." You are embarking on a forever change.

The administrator of my daughter's school once said, "There are no bad kids, just bad choices." The same truth applies to you. You were not bad today; you just made a few unwise decisions. You will make a much better selection the next time you are faced with a food choice. As you rely on God's instruction, He will let you know what and how much to eat. Your responsibility is to ask for God's assistance, make the best choice you possibly can, then pray over your decision.

To assist you in making healthy choices, I would like to share some useful tips. Over the years, I have counseled clients that if they cannot pronounce the name of an ingredient, they should not eat it. After more than a decade working in the health industry, this still proves to be a successful philosophy. In fact, with the Lord's blessing, I have employed this same strategy throughout my own recovery. Keep in mind that there are some harmful ingredients that you *can* pronounce but should still avoid. Hydrogenated oil is one such example. If you're unconvinced, I suggest that you look into the process of hydrogenation and study fact-based research on the way hydrogen solidifies in your arteries, causing dangerous plaque buildup.

I have also generally found that the fewer ingredients listed on the label, the better an item is for you. Remember, food should fuel you, so pay attention to how you feel after eating a meal. Healthy choices should cause you to feel refreshed and nourished, while poor choices often cause fatigue and bloating.

People living during New Testament times ate natural foods like goat meat, goat milk and cheese, grapes, figs, olives, honey and barley cakes, eggs, chicken, fish, beans, cucumbers, and onions. The first meal of their day was often bread made from sprouted ancient grain and cheese from a raw, unadulterated source. In the evening, they enjoyed fish, fruits, and vegetables. (I would like to point out there is no mention of Cheetos, Ho Hos, or a steroid-injected double-bacon-cheeseburger accompanied by fries and a Diet Coke.) At one time, people efficiently fueled their bodies by consuming simple, healthful meals made from fresh, whole, natural ingredients.

The key to maintaining a healthy lifestyle is to utilize a check-and-balance approach. Ask yourself if the cost of the decision outweighs the benefit. For example: Does the cost of putting that fried Twinkie in my mouth outweigh the benefits I might enjoy if I do not eat it? Are my actions causing my body more harm than good?

Maintain the mindset that, while all things are permissible, all things may not be beneficial for your body. It's your responsibility to make healthy choices. Remain steadfastly determined to apply conscientious freedom to your food selections.

Everything is permissible [allowable and lawful] for me; but not all things are helpful [good for me to do, expedient and profitable when considered with other things]. Everything is lawful for me, but I will not become the slave of anything or be brought under its power.

I Corinthians 6:12

Soul Inceptions

Reevaluate your thoughts and words so they align with your intentional purpose—becoming free from excess weight.

The fewer the ingredients listed on a food label, the better that food item is for you.

Pay attention to how you feel after eating a meal.

Chapter 11

Operation "Move It"

Taking the final step toward achieving a healthy body is not only simple, it is the most enjoyable step. The natural world of kinesiology (human movement) teaches that our bodies have two sources of stored energy: our muscles and fat. On average one pound of muscle expends a little more than sixty-five calories per day in an active individual. While stored fat burns about four calories per pound on average per day. What does this mean for you? Well, the more muscle you have, the higher your metabolism and the more energy you burn, before you even start exercising.

If you fail to provide your body with the nutritional energy it requires, it doesn't simply go without; your body will find a way to take the nutrition it needs from itself. When famished for energy, your metabolism slows down as your body searches for what it needs. It heads down the path of least resistance, straight toward your nutrient-rich muscle, which it breaks down for nourishment. To prevent this from occurring, it is important to eat every three hours.

If you wish to create a successful exercise regimen, it is critical to introduce the proper quantity of nutrients into your body. The idea is to have exercise work for you by utilizing fat for energy—and not against you by consuming muscle for energy. Understanding this process clears up the mystery of why a woman who is exercising but who only eats once a day will often plateau or perhaps even gain weight.

Types of Exercise

The only way to increase your metabolism is to increase the amount of muscle in your body. And the only way to increase muscle is to train with resistance. Resistance training is nothing more than adding resistance for your muscles to work against. This occurs during weight lifting, for example. Participating in resistance training does not mean that you will "bulk up" like a man. A woman's body has only one-fifth the amount of testosterone present in a man's body. Without high levels of testosterone and consuming a lot (I mean *a lot!*) of calories, your muscles simply can't develop the "bulky" appearance that many women prefer to avoid.

The good news is, the benefits of resistance training can be achieved through a variety of different exercise routines, including weight lifting, Pilates, using resistance bands, yoga, swimming—even carrying your children qualifies as resistance training. I'm certain that you will find a form of resistance training that appeals to you and provides results. An added benefit of resistance training is that, as your muscle fibers increase, your bone density and blood flow increase as well, while stiffness and pains in your joints will decrease.

In conjunction with resistance training, you also need to participate in cardiovascular (aerobic) exercise, which is essential for proper heart and lung health. The purpose of cardio is to improve the body's metabolic process. Simply put, the more you move, the more calories you burn. There is not a "preferred" form of cardio exercise. What do you like to do? Any movement is better than no movement at all. It makes no difference if your preference is a treadmill, elliptical trainer, stair master, using a rebounder (trampoline), or taking a cardio class. Walking, chasing the kids, cleaning the house, and dancing on Sunday during praise and worship also fall into the cardio category; **any** movement can help you achieve results. Of course, you expect to burn calories when you engage in cardio, but there are other benefits associated with this type of exercise as well, including reducing stress, eliminating toxins, and improving cardio-pulmonary efficiency.

Chapter 12

Fruits of the Spirit

Foremost, remember that your physical body should be treated no differently than any other area of your spirit-filled life. Couple your choices and actions with good spiritual truths. Be committed to mastering a new way of life. You are who you are today as a result of the choices you made yesterday, last week, and last year. Five years from now you will be who you are based on the choices you make starting today. Victory is often a process achieved by making one good choice at a time, with each and every choice supporting what you desire to achieve.

Frustration and impatience are sure signs that you are trying to achieve results in your own strength. And you've seen what your own strength can accomplish: it might get you through day three of a new exercise and nutrition regimen, but it won't sustain you to the finish line. When discouragement infiltrates your life, recognize it as a symptom that you are depending on your own strength. Ask Father God for assistance, return to the basics, and walk it out with the Fruits of the Spirit.

Fruits of the Spirit

Love. Love yourself and the body God provided for you. Your body should serve as one of your greatest allies as you carry out the mission God has ordained.

Joy. Today, I can honestly say that the last thing on my mind is food and how it may affect my weight. My focus is no longer on the food; my attention has shifted to how effective my life can become. When you keep everything in perspective, you are able to really enjoy the choices you make about what goes into your body.

> *So then, whether you eat or drink, or whatever you may do, do all for the honor and glory of God."*
>
> 1 Corinthians 10:31

Peace. You can easily become overwhelmed by the enormous amount of information that is available. Keep your eyes fixed on the Lord, and let the Holy Spirit act as your personal nutritional and strength coach. Pray over your food every time you put something in your mouth. On average, Americans encounter two hundred food choices *a day.* Pray over your choices. If there is no peace with what you are about to choose, select something else. Read and be knowledgeable about what is available and what you are eating.

Patience. Even within my prayer life, God finds opportunities to train me in patience. Keep in mind that before you can reap a harvest, there is always a season of cultivation and waiting. It is during these times that you have the opportunity to learn many important lessons. The latest diet supplement may sound enticing, but keep in mind that quick fixes are unhealthy, and their benefits are easily undone.

Kindness. Speak kindly to *your* body and speak positively of the bodies of others. Be thankful for what beautiful attributes the Lord has given to you. When you speak unkindly about yourself and meditate unfavorably on the things you do not find appealing, you are suffocating the positive attributes God intends to build upon. Make an effort to get up each morning, look at yourself in the mirror and say, *Thank you, Lord, for my smoking-hot body!* That may sound awkward at first, but the truth is that you need to change your image of yourself.

Goodness. Being "good" to yourself means that you value yourself. It also means to be of beneficial use, producing a good effect. God embodies goodness itself: "The goodness of God endureth continually.

Psalm 52:1). When God created you in His own image, He looked upon what He had made and you were *very good.*

Faith. Read the powerful promises contained in 1 Corinthians 10:13:

> *For no temptation (no trial regarded as enticing to sin), [no matter how it comes or where it leads] has overtaken you and laid hold on you that is not common to man [that is, no temptation or trial has come to you that is beyond human resistance and that is not adjusted and adapted and belonging to human experience, and such as man can bear]. But God is faithful [to His Word and to His compassionate nature], and He [can be trusted] not to let you be tempted and tried and assayed beyond your ability and strength of resistance and power to endure, but with the temptation He will [always] also provide the way out (the means of escape to a landing place), that you may be capable and strong and powerful to bear up under it patiently.*

Gentleness. Aspiring to run ten miles a day, followed by an intense forty-five-minute resistance training session may seem admirable, but it will only leave you feeling weak, fatigued, and very hungry later on. Be progressive, but increase your endurance gently, one step at a time.

Self-control. Understand that practicing self-control today has huge pay-off in the future.

> *Now every athlete who goes into training conducts himself temperately and restricts himself in all things. They do it to win a wreath that will soon wither, but we [do it to receive a crown of eternal blessedness] that cannot wither.*
>
> 1 Corinthians 9:25

Chapter 13

Conclusion: Numbers Can Do a Number on Us

Numbers go up, down, forward, and backward. There will always be greater numbers and lesser ones. Numbers are indefinite and easily manipulated. What you are truly trying to accomplish in your life can neither be measured nor conquered by the number you see on a scale, the number displayed on the tag in your jeans, or the number of calories, carbohydrates, and fat grams you consume over a specified number of hours.

As a matter of fact, numbers have a way of doing a number on you. If you allow them to, they can undermine, defeat, and humiliate. I realize that seeing a number on the scale may give you the false perception that you are "winning at life." I know, because I have lived it. In my mind, I was convinced that reaching a particular magic number would earn me a ticket into the imaginary theme park of a perfect life. The problem was, I could never do enough to achieve it. I was wasting time and energy trying to hit a moving target. The numbers were unreliable and always presented a new set of rules and variables, as numbers tend to do. The numbers are indicative of a broken system designed to hold you back from tackling the real issue—what you need to truly change from the inside out.

I've been where you may find yourself right now. I was constantly trying to measure my self-worth within the rigidity of some ridiculous, indeterminable number that I could never quantify. I was constantly exhausted, distracted, and unconvinced of my self-worth. I punished myself for the actions of others and held grudges against those who had wronged me. I was obsessed with perfection, unable to trust, and I consistently made poor decisions that were killing me. I had tried and failed too many times to count.

The journey to this point, to being able to embrace the woman I am right now, hasn't always been easy. Today, I am whole. I am able to declare this boldly because of the miracle God worked in my life—I am still alive. I am happily married to Esteban, an amazing man; I am blessed to be called "Mom" by my two terrific children, Olivia and Angelo. My life has been completely restored, and, because of my past challenges and triumphs, I have a heart for women who struggle with body image. I have a passion to see you live in complete freedom with food.

If food is a challenge, you are bearing a burden you were never meant to carry. God desires for you to lay down this weight at His feet and allow Him to develop you into the incredible person He designed. I invite you to spend some time in prayerful meditation before Father God. Discover the future He has planned for you. Accept His grace and compassion for you as the unique, wonderful, passionate, beautiful, talented woman of God that is His creation. Read over the letter of commitment on the next page. Sign it when you're ready. Post it where you can refer to it often. Commit yourself and your choices to God every day and before every meal. Isn't it time you committed to doing what's best for you so that you can live your best life through Christ?

A Letter of Commitment

Sweet Father God:

I no longer come to You out of fear of my lost battle with weight. I no longer come to You out of fear of disease and illness. Today I accept and receive the gift of strength You have given me. I no longer accept defeat. Instead, I commit to Your will with the knowledge that I have Your never-ending support.

I am ready, Lord, to let go of unrealistic demands and images. I am ready to respect my body and care for it, no longer taking it for granted. I will always remember that You sent me into the world with this body, and I commit to caring for it as a most precious gift. I am ready to accept responsibility for acquiring a healthy body because You have a purpose for me to accomplish in this life. You have gifts for me to share, as well as a legacy to leave for all of those who will come after me. Discarding past frustrations, I commit myself to You today. I set goals out of love, joy, peace, patience, kindness, goodness, faith, gentleness, and self-control; the very fruits of Your Spirit. In Jesus's Name, I pray. Amen.

Signed:
Dated:

Notes

Chapter 2: Going On

Brainy Quote, "Ben Franklin Quotes (Benjamin Franklin Quotes)," Copyright 2009 Brainy Media.com, http://www.brainyquote.com/quotes/authors/b/ben_franklin.html

Chapter 3: Satan's Tools of Self-Sabotage

1. Centers for Disease Control and Prevention, "New CDC Study Finds No Increase in Obesity Among Adults; But Levels Still High," *NCHS Press Room,* November 28, 2007, http://www.cdc.gov/nchs/pressroom/07newsrelease/obesity.htm (accessed June 11, 2009).
2. Centers for Disease Control and Prevention, "Prevalence of Overweight Among Children and Adolescents: United States 2003–2004," *NCHS Health and Stats, April* 2006, http://www.cdc.gov/nchs/products/pubd/hestats/overweight/overwght_child_03.htm (accessed September 09, 2008).
3. National Association of Anorexia Nervosa and Associated Disorders (ANAD), Facts About Eating Disorders, http://www.anad.org/2285/index.html
4. Leah Hoffman and Lacey Rose, "Costly calories, how much do we spend on diets," http://www.msnbc.msn.com/id/7432448/ns/health-fitness/t/costly-calories (accessed April 13, 2005).

5. Kevin Stirtz, "Remarkable Service Starts with a Great First Impression," http://www.americanchronicle.com/articles/view/49179 (accessed January 15, 2008).

Chapter 9: Reevaluating Fixations

1. Answer Fitness: Practical Fitness Advice For Everyone, "How Many Calories Should I Eat To Lose Weight: Ask The Fitness Nerd" http://www.answerfitness.com/212/how-many-calories-eat-lose-weight/ (accessed December 24, 2008).
2. Peter Bennett, N.D., *The Purification Plan*, 161–162.
3. Ibid., 339.